Nutrition FUN with Brocc & Roll

A Hands-On Activity Guide Filled with Delicious Learning!

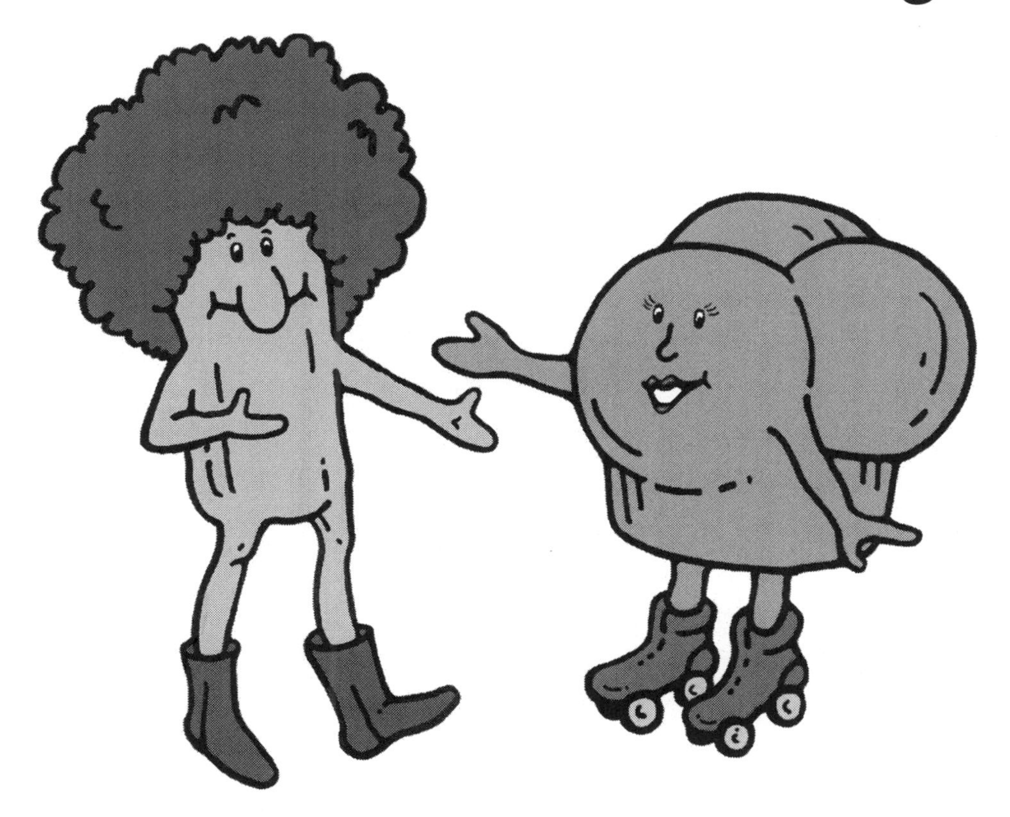

Connie Liakos Evers, MS, RD

24 Carrot Press ♦ Portland, Oregon

24 Carrot Press
PO Box 23546
Portland, OR 97281
503-524-9318
www.nutritionforkids.com

Nutrition Fun with Brocc & Roll, 2nd edition

Cover, design and illustration: Carol Buckle, www.cjbuckle.com

Printed in the United States of America

ISBN: 978-0-9647970-9-3

More books by Connie Liakos Evers, MS, RD
How to Teach Nutrition to Kids, 4th edition (24 Carrot Press, ©2012)
Good for You! Nutrition Book and Games (Disney Press, ©2006)

For updates, free resources and more, visit us online:
www.nutritionforkids.com
www.facebook.com/nutritionforkids
twitter.com/nutritionkids

TABLE OF CONTENTS

Introduction **5**
How to Use This Guide: Notes to Educators 5
Suggested Grade Levels 5
Evaluation 5
Notes to Parents 6
What Kids Need to Know 7
Making the Connection: Food Gives Me Energy (worksheet) 8

Chapter 1: Self-Assessment **9**
Sizing up My Diet 10
MyPlate 10
Pocket Tally 12
Nutrition Abacus 14
What's My Serving Size? 15
MyPlate: What Kids Need to Eat Each Day 16
Breakfast Cereal/Spaghetti 17
100% Fruit Juice/Cheese 18
Weekly Activity Tally 19
My Body Is a Great Body! 20

Chapter 2: Setting Goals and Making Choices **21**
Goal Setting 23
Goal-Setting Calendar 24
My Goals for Good Health 26
Bravo for Breakfast! 27
Make a Snack Plan 28
A Role-Playing Game: Thinking Through Our Choices 29

Chapter 3: Finding out More About the Food You Eat **31**
Label Logic 32
Are You a Food Fact Finder? 32
Potatoes 33
Breakfast Bars 34
Be an Ad-Buster 35
Analyzing "Frooty-Tooty Fruitsies" 35
A Closer Look at Saturday Morning TV 36
Not so Fast...Make a Game Plan for Eating Out 37

Chapter 4: Cooking Up Some Fun! **39**
Wacky Snacks 40
Make Your Own Recipes 42
Egg-Xactly Right Eggs 42
Fuel-Up Trail Mix 43
Perfectly Personal Pizza 44
Soup Like You Like It 45
Stir-Fry Surprise 46
Recipe Review 47

Chapter 5: Growing Fun **49**
Get Started in the Garden (Checklist) 50
Keep a Garden Journal 51
Plant a Theme Garden 52
Grow an Indoor Herb Garden 53
Discover Food Where You live 54

Chapter 6: Puzzles, Activities and More Recipes **55**
Use Your Brain to Find Whole Grains 57
Veggie Plant Parts 58
Fruit: Nature's Sweet Treats 59
The Protein Scene 60
A *M-O-O-O-O-VING* Story About Dairy 61
A Month of Fitness & Fun! Calendar 63
It's Hugh-Man (and the Foodettes) Puppet Page 64

ABOUT THE SPOKES-FOODS...

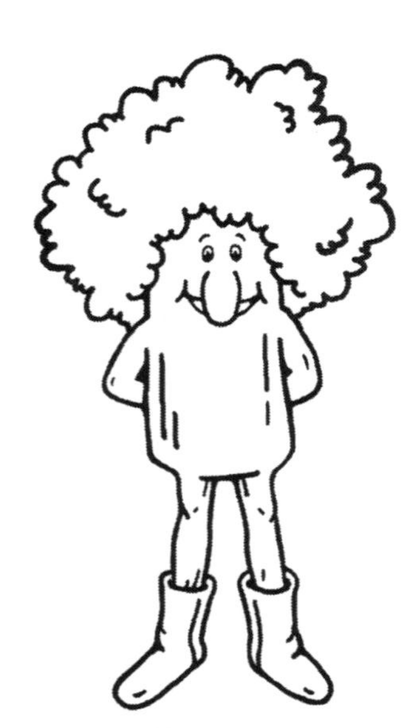

Brocc

Brocc lives in a beautiful, green field near Salinas, California.

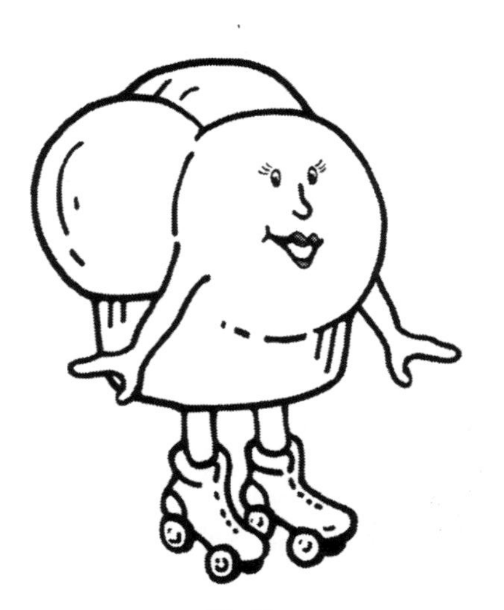

Roll

Strictly a whole-grain kind of girl, Roll's family originated in a Kansas wheat field.

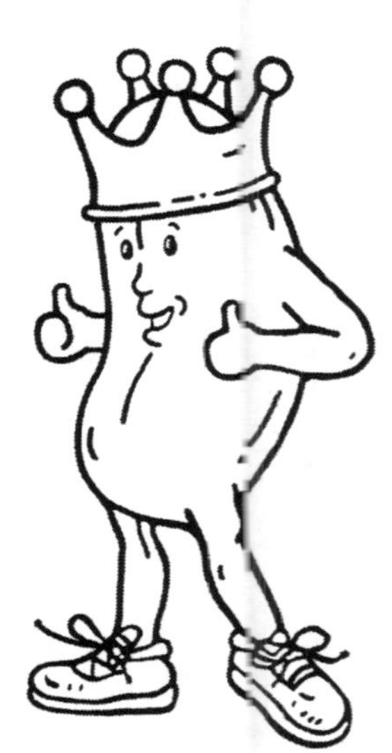

Hugh-Man Bean

A human be-an Hugh-Man is a kidney bean who resides in the Red River Valley of Minnesota.

INTRODUCTION

The overall goal of *Nutrition Fun with Brocc & Roll* is to make the study of food and nutrition engaging and relevant for today's children. This guide combines a discovery approach to learning with a healthy dose of humor. Important life skills are gained when kids learn to assess food and activity habits, set goals, make choices, understand advertising and label reading, learn to plan and develop basic cooking skills. A chapter on "Growing Fun" helps children to more fully understand the "roots" of the food they eat each day.

HOW TO USE THIS GUIDE: Notes to Educators

Nutrition Fun with Brocc & Roll is designed to be used in conjunction with the book *How to Teach Nutrition to Kids,* 4th ed., which includes background information about nutrition, tips on how to promote positive messages, the importance of making nutrition fun, and more than 200 activities to help you implement these concepts. You can order *How to Teach Nutrition to Kids* online at www.nutritionforkids.com.

***Brocc & Roll* can be used in the following ways:**

- As you are planning your nutrition and health curricula, this guide will provide you with structure, sequence and hands-on activities.
- Many of the lesson ideas in this guide work well as stand-alone activities that you can teach throughout the year as a reinforcement for healthful eating and as a way to integrate nutrition concepts into your curriculum. For example, in Chapter 2 students learn the importance of goal setting, a skill that transfers to study habits and other areas of life. In Chapter 3, they explore advertising from a food point of view, an important complement to a unit on media literacy.
- *Brocc & Roll* also provides many ideas for food and nutrition lessons that can be used during special events and celebrations such as wellness week, National Nutrition Month®, National School Breakfast or Lunch Week, heart month and health fairs.

SUGGESTED GRADE LEVELS

The copy-ready masters include information on the bottom of the page regarding suggested elementary grade levels. These are not carved-in-stone levels, but simply guidelines to help you when planning lessons. You will find that many of the activities reach beyond these age ranges, and some may be adaptable for early childhood or the middle school grade levels.

EVALUATION

A common question among nutrition educators is, "How do I know that I am making a difference?" Oftentimes, children may learn a great deal about food and nutrition but fail to put their new-found wisdom into practice. The self-assessment activities in Chapter 1 provide the cornerstone for evaluating behavior change. It is recommended that children repeat the food and activity assessments found in Chapter 1 throughout the school year. This provides a way to measure and observe change over time.

NOTES TO PARENTS

Author's note: I have included this short section for parents because I have found that many parents use this guide to teach their own children and/or serve as scouting or group leaders. In addition, many of the educators and health professionals who use this guide work with parents on a regular basis.

If you are serious about getting your kids to eat right and move more, there are a few "beans" of wisdom that you need to know. These are common sense guidelines, yet they make all the difference in helping your children form healthful, lifelong eating habits.

- Be a role model for healthful eating. Children really do learn best by example.
- Make family meals a priority. Not only do children form better food habits, but it is also a great opportunity for strengthening family relationships. Children who grow up with family meals are often better adjusted and less prone to risky behavior as teens.

"Listen up for some leguminous advice."

- Buy mostly healthful foods that follow the recommendations of the *MyPlate* food guidance system. There's nothing wrong with occasional treats and sweets, but the core of the diet should consist of whole grains, whole fruits, vegetables, lean protein foods, seafood and fat-free or low-fat dairy products.
- Breakfast is the meal most directly linked with academic achievement, focus and learning. There is also research that suggests breakfast eaters have an easier time achieving a healthy weight. To plan an optimal breakfast, use my "rule of 3" which includes a protein source (from protein or dairy group), a serving of whole grain and a serving of either fruit or vegetable.
- Improve your family's health and save money by drinking water when thirsty. Limit sugary beverages and restrict 100% fruit juice to just 4-8 ounces/day. Serve nutrient-rich low-fat or fat-free milk with meals and snacks.
- Promote healthy eating development by letting children serve themselves at the table. Never force children to eat a certain amount or clean their plates. Allow kids to respond to their own feelings of hunger and fullness.
- Monitor and limit "screen time" (television, movies, mobile devices, touchscreen tablets and computers). A good goal for school-aged children is a maximum of 2 hours of non-educational screen time each day.
- Every day, children should engage in at least one hour of moderate to vigorous physical activity such as P.E., organized sports or active play. Encourage a balance of activities, including plenty of time for good ol' outside play.

WHAT KIDS NEED TO KNOW

Emphasize food as it relates to life today.

◆ You will lose kids' attention faster than they can say "osteoporosis" if too much emphasis is placed on how proper nutrition prevents disease. If you succeed in reaching them with the good nutrition message today, their tomorrows will likely be healthier too.

◆ Remind children that healthful food promotes achievement. In school or on the playing field, kids who eat well perform better and achieve higher levels of mastery. A nutritious diet fuels the body for learning, growth, sports and play.

◆ A fun way to introduce this concept is to use the "Food gives me energy..." sheet on page 8. This activity helps children make the connection between healthy eating and how it gives them the energy needed to participate in the activities that they most enjoy.

The message of good nutrition is summed up in the *Dietary Guidelines for Americans.*

◆ Adults and kids over the age of two are advised to balance their diets by eating from a wide selection of foods, emphasizing fruits, vegetables, whole grains, lean protein, seafood and fat-free or low-fat dairy foods; and to choose sensibly by moderating the amount of trans and saturated fat, added sugars and sodium they eat.

◆Two important practical tools for meeting these guidelines are the *MyPlate* food guide and the *Nutrition Facts* food label.

Teach children to refuel their bodies!

◆ Because of their smaller stomach capacity and tremendous energy needs, kids require regular meals and snacks. Behavior problems at times are merely the result of an empty stomach.

◆ Breakfast is the meal most directly connected to school achievement. Kids who skip breakfast have shorter attention spans, do poorly in tasks requiring concentration and even score lower on standard achievement tests.

◆ Somehow, "snacking" has taken on a negative connotation in our society, perhaps because it is often linked with low-nutrient foods. Done right, snacks can and do make a big contribution to daily nutrition. Healthful snacks should mirror meals – emphasizing healthful foods, but in smaller quantities.

Young bodies need to move!

◆ Kids should be getting at least one hour of moderate to vigorous physical activity each day. Physical fitness should also be part of recess and the daily classroom routine, especially in schools that limit PE to once or twice weekly.

Media literacy should be a part of every child's education.

◆ If children are to resist the allure of the media, advertisements and other societal influences, they must learn to critically analyze and evaluate the source and intent of media messages.

Source: ***How to Teach Nutrition to Kids, 4th ed.*** pages 26–29

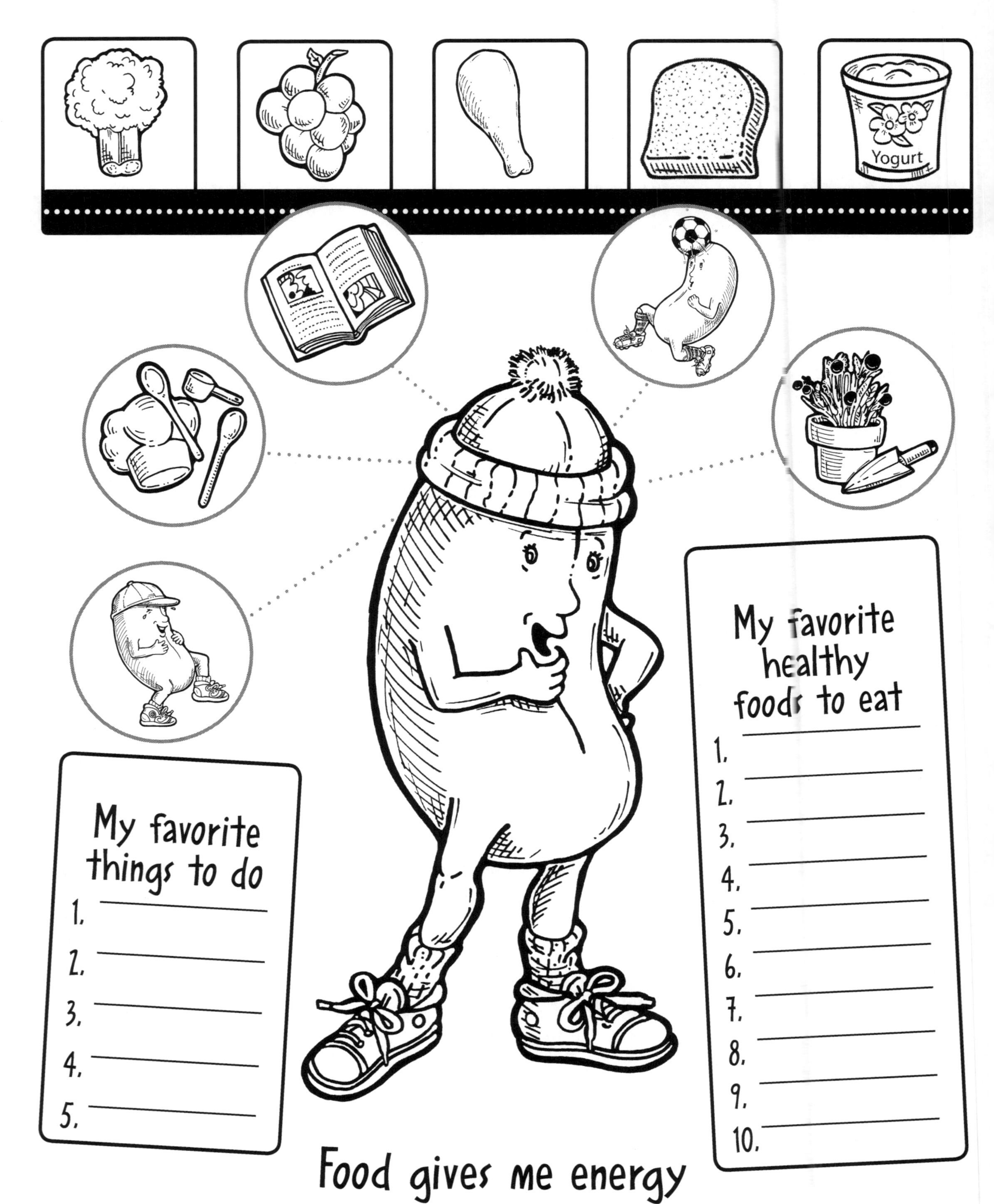

Food gives me energy
So I can do...MY FAVORITE THINGS! How about you?

Suggested Level: K–2nd grade

SELF-ASSESSMENT

NOTES TO EDUCATORS

The activities in this chapter form the basis of evaluating the effectiveness of your nutrition education unit.

◆ Begin your nutrition unit by having the children track their eating habits for three to seven days using one or more of the methods outlined in this chapter. Children have three options for tracking their daily eating habits: ***MyPlate,*** the **Pocket Tally** or the **Nutrition Abacus**.

The serving size activities on pages 15–18 will aid children in better gauging the number of servings that they are actually eating.

Encourage children to complete the **Weekly Activity Tally** for one week. Stress the important relationship between food and activity and the importance of being active at least **one hour** each day.

◆ Today's children are becoming increasingly obsessed about their body shape and size, developing unhealthy attitudes that may lead to disordered eating (for a discussion of this issue, please see pages 22–26 in *How to Teach Nutrition to Kids*). **My Body Is a Great Body!** is an activity sheet designed to help children identify their strengths and contribute to a healthier body image. In conjunction with this activity, discuss how bodies come in a wide variety of shapes and sizes and how everyone grows and develops at different rates.

IN THIS CHAPTER:

Sizing Up My Diet
MyPlate
Pocket Tally
Nutrition Abacus
What's My Serving Size?
Notes to Educators
MyPlate: What Kids Need to Eat Each Day
Breakfast Cereal/Spaghetti
100% Fruit Juice/Cheese
Weekly Activity Tally
My Body Is a Great Body!

◆ For the duration of the nutrition unit, students should continue to monitor and track their progress. As they learn more about nutrition and fitness and set goals for their personal health, these self-monitoring activities will allow them to visually chart their progress over time.

◆ During the school year, children should periodically be encouraged to reassess their food and activity behavior.

◆ This is also a great homework activity that can involve the entire family in assessing diet and activity patterns.

◆ Teachers and adult leaders will also benefit from tracking eating and exercise habits. Setting a good example is a powerful reinforcer for children.

SIZING UP MY DIET

MyPlate

Name ______________________

DIRECTIONS

1. Make copies of the blank *MyPlate* on page 11. Use one sheet for each day that you keep track of your diet.
2. Each time you eat or drink, write the name and amount of each food and beverage in the correct food group space on *MyPlate* (you can also draw a picture of each food if you prefer).
3. The *MyPlate: What Kids Need to Eat Each Day* chart on page 16 will help if you have questions about where to record your foods. If you eat a mixed food such as a vegetable burrito, you will record the tortilla in the grains group, the vegetables in the vegetables group, the cheese in the dairy group and the beans in the protein group.
4. Record any "extra" foods such as candy, chocolate, cookies, doughnuts, sweetened drinks or fried chips in the box below the blank *MyPlate*.
5. At the end of each day, compare your *MyPlate* to the recommendations from the chart on page 16 or information from the www.choosemyplate.gov website. Then answer the following questions.

QUESTIONS

1. Check your record for balance:

   Did you eat something from every food group? ______________________

   ____

   List any groups with fewer than the suggested servings. ______________________

   ____

   List any groups with more than the suggested servings. ______________________

   ____

2. Was today a "normal" day? Was there anything that happened today that changed your eating habits? ______________________

   ____

3. Are there changes you could make to better balance your *MyPlate*? ______________________

   ____

Did you know that you may not need to eat exactly everything *MyPlate* tells you to? Just as we have different hair, eyes and favorite activities, we also have different nutrition needs. For example, you may need more food or less food than *MyPlate* suggests. Some families don't eat certain foods because of their beliefs or religion. Other times, allergies or medical conditions affect the foods that you can eat. Remember – *MyPlate* is only a guide!

Name: ______________________ Date: ______________________

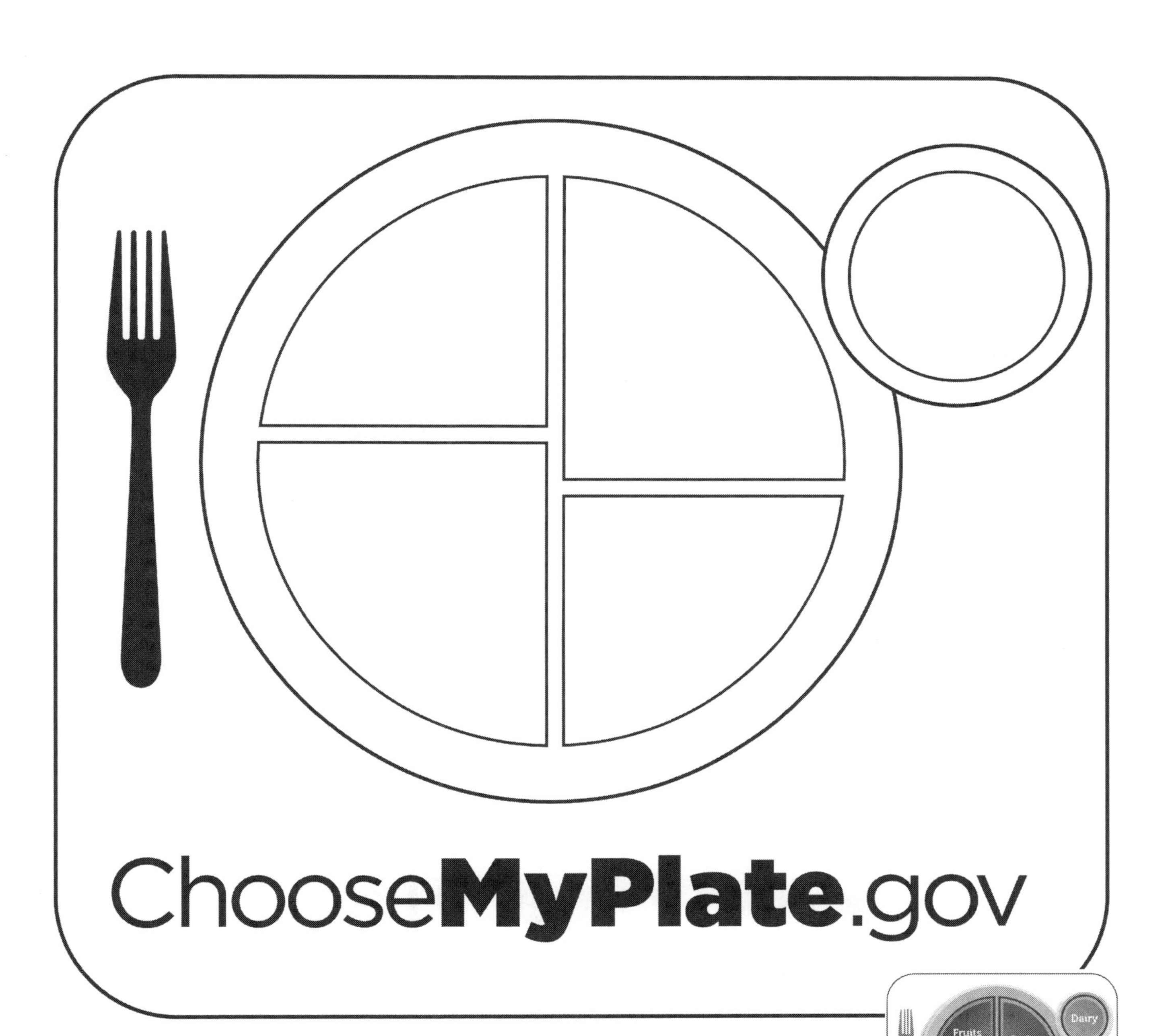

Extra foods* I ate today:

____

____

Fruits
Grains
Dairy
Vegetables
Protein
ChooseMyPlate.gov

*Extra foods include high-calorie, low-nutrition choices such as candy, chocolate, cookies, doughnuts, sweetened drinks and fried chips. Try to limit these to a maximum of one to two servings on most days.

Suggested Level: 3rd–6th grade

SIZING UP MY DIET

Pocket Tally

DIRECTIONS

1. Cut out the pocket tallies on the next page. Staple them together and put them in a handy place so you will remember to record what you eat.
2. Each time you eat or drink, write the name of the food or beverage on your pocket record. Next, place a tally mark in the correct food group. For example, if you had cereal, yogurt and juice for breakfast, place tally marks in the Grains, Dairy and Fruits groups.
   • The *MyPlate: What Kids Need to Eat Each Day* chart on page 16 will help you to decide where to place foods and calculate the number of servings in the food group categories.
   • At the end of each day, answer the questions at the bottom of this page.

EXAMPLE ➡

MY POCKET TALLY

Name Brocc Greenfield Date March 10, 2012

What I ate today:	Vegetables	Fruits	Grains	Dairy	Protein	Extras
Breakfast: 1 whole-wheat tortilla, 1 scrambled egg, 1 slice cheese, 1 cup orange juice		I	I	I	I	
Lunch: 1 turkey sandwich*, carrot sticks, apple, 1 carton 1% milk	I	I	II	I	II	
Dinner: 1 piece chicken & rice, salad w/ranch, 1 serving asparagus, 2 cookies	II		I		III	II
Snacks: 1 banana, 1 carton blueberry yogurt, 2 whole-grain crackers, 2 more cookies		I	I	I		I
Totals:	3	3	5	3	6oz	3

*Turkey breast on sandwich is approximately 2 ounces; chicken breast is approximately 3 ounces

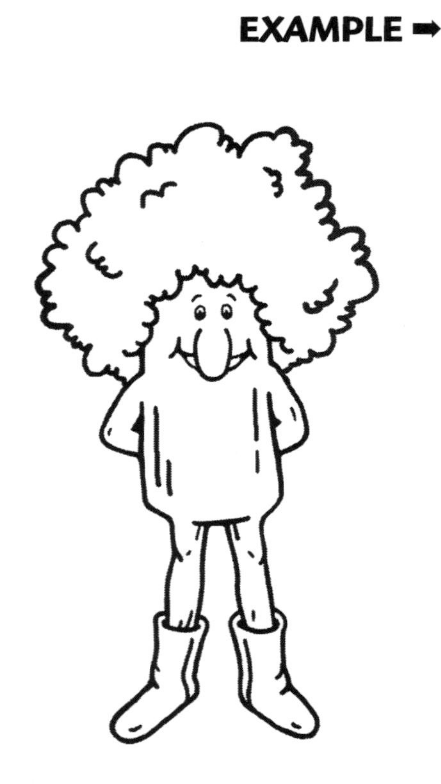

HOW DID I DO TODAY?

1. Did I eat breakfast?
2. Did I eat the suggested number of servings from each group?
3. Did I make progress on a personal nutrition goal?

   Explain ______________________________

   ____

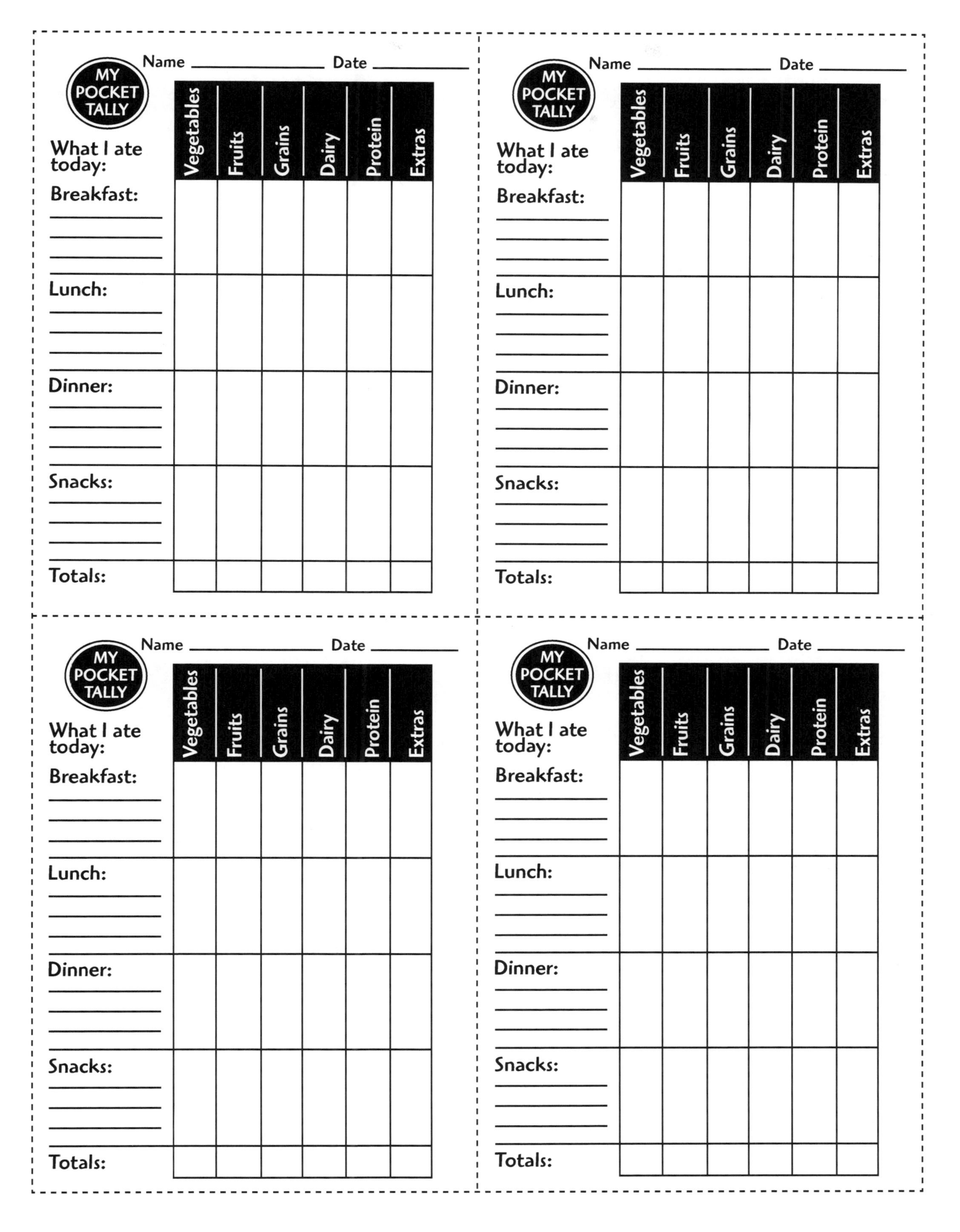
MY POCKET TALLY

Name ______________ Date __________

What I ate today:	Vegetables	Fruits	Grains	Dairy	Protein	Extras
Breakfast:						
Lunch:						
Dinner:						
Snacks:						
Totals:						

MY POCKET TALLY

Name ______________ Date __________

What I ate today:	Vegetables	Fruits	Grains	Dairy	Protein	Extras
Breakfast:						
Lunch:						
Dinner:						
Snacks:						
Totals:						

MY POCKET TALLY

Name ______________ Date __________

What I ate today:	Vegetables	Fruits	Grains	Dairy	Protein	Extras
Breakfast:						
Lunch:						
Dinner:						
Snacks:						
Totals:						

MY POCKET TALLY

Name ______________ Date __________

What I ate today:	Vegetables	Fruits	Grains	Dairy	Protein	Extras
Breakfast:						
Lunch:						
Dinner:						
Snacks:						
Totals:						

SIZING UP MY DIET

Nutrition Abacus

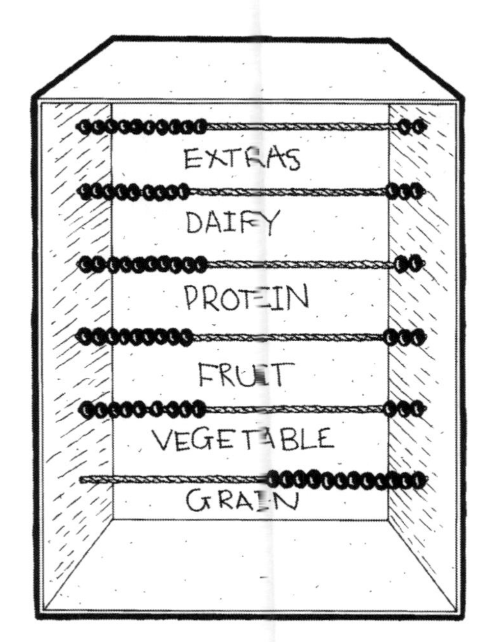

YOU WILL NEED

Shoe box

String or twine

72 buttons or beads (in six different colors, if possible)

markers or crayons

DIRECTIONS

1. Write the names of the food groups on the bottom of the box as shown in the picture. The groups are Grains, Vegetables, Fruits, Dairy, Protein and Extras.
2. Punch six small holes along one of the long sides of the shoe box. Punch six more on the other side that pair up with the first set of holes.
3. Cut six pieces of string that are approximately twice the width of the box.
4. Knot each piece of string on one side and thread through the holes. Feed 12 beads or buttons onto each string.
5. Thread the string through the opposite hole, and tie a knot on the end to secure.

Once you have completed your **Nutrition Abacus**, use it to check your daily food habits:

- Each time you eat a meal or snack, move a bead across for every serving that you eat from each food group. By the end of the day, you can see if the beads that you moved across match the guidelines of *MyPlate* listed on page 16. HINT: It may be easier to use the **Nutrition Abacus** once you have recorded your diet using ***MyPlate*** or **Pocket Tally**.
- The **Nutrition Abacus** is also a great planning tool. Use it to check if the school menu, your after-school snack or your favorite meals are "*MyPlate* balanced."

Did you know that you may not need to eat exactly everything *MyPlate* tells you to? Just as we have different hair, eyes and favorite activities, we also have different nutrition needs. For example, you may need more food or less food than *MyPlate* suggests. Some families don't eat certain foods because of their beliefs or religion. Other times, allergies or medical conditions affect the foods that you can eat. Remember – *MyPlate* is only a guide!

WHAT'S MY SERVING SIZE?

NOTES TO EDUCATORS

- The activities on pages 17 and 18 will help you and the students to understand serving sizes referenced by *MyPlate*. It doesn't mean that everyone has to eat this exact amount. But it is critical to understand the concept of how much a serving is if you are trying to accurately track your diet.
- Most children need to eat at least the minimum number of servings for proper nutrition. But many kids will need more, especially those who are active in sports and play. Discuss with children the importance of "listening" to their bodies to tell them how much to eat. Ask the children how it feels to eat too much, not enough and just the right amount. For a complete discussion of this issue, including the use of a hunger scale, refer to pages 48-49 in *How to Teach Nutrition to Kids.*
- The serving size activities are best set up as "measuring centers." Hands-on experience measuring foods will give children a better grasp of what a serving really looks like.
- Since everyone is touching the foods, caution the children that this is NOT an eating activity. You may want to plan this activity in conjunction with a snack or conduct it right after lunch.
- For more ideas on measuring centers for additional foods, please refer to page 57 in the book *How to Teach Nutrition to Kids.*

SUPPLIES NEEDED

Measuring cups (dry and liquid)

Food scale or gram scale

Waxed paper

Serving utensils

Plates and bowls

Drinking glasses (a variety of sizes, if desired)

Cooked pasta (soak in water beforehand to avoid sticking)

Box of ready-to-eat cereal

100% fruit juice

Cheese (cubes, slices and/or grated)

MyPlate: WHAT KIDS NEED TO EAT EACH DAY*

FOOD GROUP	AMOUNT NEEDED EACH DAY	EXAMPLES & SERVING SIZES	GO EASY ON:
Grains	5 to 7 ounces (at least half from whole grain sources)	1 ounce is approximately: 1 slice of bread; 1 cup of dry cereal; 1/2 cup of rice, pasta or cooked cereal; 3 cups of popcorn; 1 small tortilla; 7 round crackers	Refined grains and grains with added sugars
Vegetables	1-1/2 to 2-1/2 cups	1 cup cooked or chopped vegetables; 2 cups salad greens is considered 1 cup from the vegetable group (Emphasize colorful veggies)	High-fat salad dressings, butter added to cooked vegetables and fried vegetables such as French fries
Fruits	1-1/2 cups to 2 cups	1 cup of fruit or 8 ounces of 100% juice **Also equal to 1 cup of fruit:** 1 small apple; 1 large banana; 1 large orange; 32 grapes; 1/2 cup dried fruit	Fruit with added sugar Limit fruit juice to 4-8 oz. daily
Dairy	2.5 cups (ages 4 to 8) 3 cups (age 9 & older)	1 cup of milk or yogurt or 1-1/2 ounces of cheese; 1 cup calcium-fortified soymilk	High-fat cheeses and high-sugar dairy desserts
Protein	4 to 6 ounces total of meat or meat equivalents	1 ounce lean meat, poultry or seafood; 1/4 cup beans; 1 egg; 1 tablespoon of peanut butter; 1/2 ounce (about 2 tablespoons) of shelled sunflower seeds or nuts	High-fat and/or cured meats, poultry with the skin left on and fried protein foods

Limit "Extra" foods such as candy, chocolate, cookies, donuts, sweetened drinks and fried chips to no more than 1 to 2 servings on most days.

*These are general guidelines for a 6-11 year-old child's daily food intake. For a personalized *Daily Food Plan* based on age, gender, height, weight and activity level visit www.choosemyplate.gov. The *MyPlate* site also provides more detailed information on serving sizes.

WHAT'S YOUR SERVING SIZE OF CEREAL?

Name ___________________________

DIRECTIONS

1. Pretend it is breakfast time and you are hungry for your favorite cereal.
2. Using a cereal bowl, pour in the amount that you normally would eat for breakfast.
3. Using a 1/4 cup measuring cup, measure how many scoops of cereal you just poured into your bowl. What is the total amount in your bowl? ________
4. Look at the *Nutrition Facts* label on the cereal box. What is the serving size? ________
5. How many servings did you pour into your bowl? ________

It's normal to eat more than one serving of a food group at one meal. The *MyPlate* food guidance system encourages kids to eat 5 to 7 ounces daily servings from the grain group. At least half of your grains should be from whole grain sources. The reason for this activity is to give you a better idea of how to keep track of your servings each day.

✂- -

WHAT'S YOUR SERVING SIZE OF SPAGHETTI?

Name ___________________________

DIRECTIONS

1. Pretend it is dinnertime and your family is serving spaghetti.
2. Using a dinner plate, scoop up the amount of spaghetti that you normally would eat for dinner.
3. Using a 1/2 cup measuring cup, measure how many 1/2 cup scoops of spaghetti that you just placed on your plate. What is the total amount on your plate? ________
4. Look at the *Nutrition Facts* label on the spaghetti package or refer to the chart on page 16. What is the serving size for spaghetti (pasta)? ________
5. How many servings did you place on your plate? ________

It's normal to eat more than one serving of a food group at one meal. The *MyPlate* food guidance system encourages kids to eat 5 to 7 ounces daily servings from the grain group. At least half of your grains should be from whole grain sources. The reason for this activity is to give you a better idea of how to keep track of your servings each day.

Suggested Level: 1st - 6th grade

WHAT'S YOUR SERVING SIZE OF 100% FRUIT JUICE?

Name ____________________________

DIRECTIONS

1. Pretend you are thirsty for a glass of 100% fruit juice.
2. Using a drinking glass, pour in the amount that you normally would drink.
3. Using a liquid measuring cup, measure how many ounces of juice that you just poured into your glass. How many ounces are in your glass? ________
4. Look at the *Nutrition Facts* label on the juice container or refer to the chart on page 16. What is the serving size for 100% fruit juice? ________
5. How many servings did you pour into your glass? ________

Whenever possible, it's better to choose whole fruit instead of fruit juice. Try to limit juice to 4–8 ounces per day. The *MyPlate* food guidance system encourages kids to eat 1½ to 2 cups of fruit daily. The reason for this activity is to give you a better idea of how to keep track of your servings each day.

✂- -

WHAT'S YOUR SERVING SIZE OF CHEESE?

Name ____________________________

DIRECTIONS

1. Pretend it is snack time and you are hungry for whole-grain crackers and cheese.
2. Choose the amount of cheese that you would normally eat for your snack.
3. Place your cheese on a sheet of waxed paper and place on the food or gram scale. How many ounces does your cheese weigh? ________
4. Look at the *Nutrition Facts* label on the cheese package or refer to the chart on page 16. What is the serving size for cheese? ________
5. How many servings did you choose? ________

The *MyPlate* food guidance system encourages kids to consume 3 cups of dairy (or foods made from dairy) daily. A serving is 1 cup of milk or yogurt, 1-1/2 ounces of cheese, or 1 cup of calcium-fortified soymilk. The reason for this activity is to give you a better idea of how to keep track of your servings each day.

WEEKLY ACTIVITY TALLY

Name ______________________________

"Gotta run. The chef's cooking bean cuisine today!"

"And I don't want to be a has-bean."

Are you an active, busy kid full of energy? Or do you sit too much in front of the television or computer? Every day, we have to sit still part of the day (in school) and our bodies also need to rest (at night).

• Other times, though, our bodies need to MOVE. Not only does moving our bodies work our muscles, strengthen our heart and keep us healthy, it can also be a whole lot of FUN!

• It is important to be active for at least **one hour** every single day. Keep track of your activities this week. Keep a tally of how many times you participate in an activity and also how many total minutes that you spend in this activity.

AEROBIC* ACTIVITIES

Try for at least *five* each week

___Biking ___ minutes ___In-line Skating ___ minutes ___Dancing ___ minutes

___Fast Walking ___ minutes ___Cross-Country Skiing ___ minutes ___Jumping Rope ___ minutes

___Running ___ minutes ___Hiking ___ minutes ___Swimming ___ minutes

________________ minutes: ____ ________________ minutes: ____ ________________ minutes: ____

*Aerobic activities are those that you can do at a steady pace for at least **15 minutes**. You should be breathing a little hard, but you *should not* feel out of breath.

TOTAL AEROBIC ACTIVITIES _______

TOTAL AEROBIC MINUTES _______

GAMES & SPORTS

Try for at least two to three each week

___ Tag ___ minutes ___ Basketball ___ minutes ___ Soccer ___ minutes

___ Volleyball___ minutes ___ Wall Ball ___ minutes ___ Football ___ minutes

___ Ice Skating ___ minutes ___ Gymnastics ___ minute ___ Karate or Tae Kwon Do ___ minutes

________________ minutes: ____ ________________ minutes: ____ ________________ minutes: ____

TOTAL GAMES & SPORTS _______

TOTAL GAMES & SPORTS MINUTES _______

OTHER WORK & PLAY ACTIVITIES

Try for at least two to three each week

___ Chores ___ minutes ___ Gardening ___ minutes ___ Bowling ___ minutes

___ Golf ___ minutes ___ Hopscotch ___ minutes ___ Stretching ___ minutes

___ Tetherball ___ minutes

________________ minutes: ____ ________________ minutes: ____ ________________ minutes: ____

TOTAL MINUTES OF ACTIVITY THIS WEEK _______
AVERAGE DAILY MINUTES THIS WEEK _______
(Divide the number above by 7)

TOTAL WORK & PLAY ACTIVITIES _______

TOTAL WORK & PLAY MINUTES _______

Suggested Level: 3rd - 6th grade

MY BODY IS A GREAT BODY!

Name ____________________________

Did you know that *every* body is a great body? Bodies come in a wide variety of colors, shapes and sizes. Some of us are taller, shorter, rounder or thinner. The one thing we do all have in common is the choice to take the best care of our very own, very great body!

Fill in the blanks below about your great body:

- The thing I like best about my body is ____________________
- My body is good at ____________________
- When my body feels rested and energetic, I like to ____________________
- When my body feels quiet and less energetic, I like to ____________________

Some of the ways I take care of my body:

1. ____________________
2. ____________________
3. ____________________
4. ____________________
5. ____________________

"Rolling along and singing a song. That keeps my body happy and strong."

A PICTURE OF MY GREAT BODY:

Suggested Level: 1st - 6th grade

SETTING GOALS AND MAKING CHOICES

NOTES TO EDUCATORS

Our job as nutrition educators and parents is to provide kids with the opportunity and knowledge to make healthful choices. Sometimes though, in spite of our best efforts, we observe children who make mostly poor food choices. Frustrated, we may blame ourselves for failing to properly educate children about nutrition.

IN THIS CHAPTER:

Goal Setting
- Goal-Setting Calendar
- My Goals for Good Health

Bravo for Breakfast!
Make a Snack Plan
Role-Playing Game: Thinking Through Our Choices

But while we can offer nutrition experiences that reinforce good eating habits, provide mostly healthful food choices, and model good eating practices, the decision to put nutrition knowledge into practice ultimately lies with each *individual child.*

In this chapter you will find activities that empower children by allowing them to set and monitor goals, make their own plans for breakfast and snack time, and role play the choices they would make in a variety of situations. In other words, the activities presented here reinforce the control that children have over their own health and nutrition.

GOAL SETTING FOR THE PRIMARY LEVEL

For younger children, the worksheet on page 26 is an introduction to goal setting. Explain to children that a goal is like a plan. Just as plans are sometimes changed or interrupted, goals may need to be modified in order to achieve success.

Setting goals is something children can apply to many areas of their life, including academics, behavior, physical fitness, nutrition and other areas of health. Parents and teachers can serve as role models by setting good health goals along with the children.

SETTING S.N.A.C.K. GOALS

Intermediate students can begin to set more specific goals that can be quantified and measured. The S.N.A.C.K. system allows the child to set effective goals that are more likely to prove successful. Encourage students to evaluate their goals to make sure they meet the criteria of S.N.A.C.K. listed on page 22.

S.N.A.C.K. GOALS

S = Small

Is this goal small enough so I can meet it in a short period of time?

N = Needed

Is this a change that I need to make for better health?

A = Achievable

Can I achieve this goal? Will I need the help of others to meet this goal? Is it a goal that I can really accomplish?

C = Can I Count It?

Is this goal written in a way that I can count and measure my progress?

K = Know-How

Do I know enough to set this health goal? Where would I find more information on this topic?

GOAL SETTING

"I know how to score a goal, but how do you *set* a goal?"

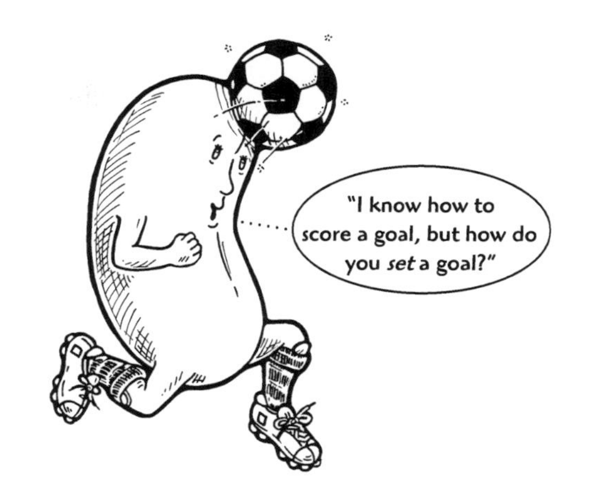

Have you sized up your diet yet using *MyPlate*, the *Pocket Tally* or the *Nutrition Abacus*? Have you completed the *Weekly Activity Tally*? If so, you may have noticed a few changes you could make to improve your health habits.

Whenever you want to make a change, the first thing you need to do is to set a goal. A great way to succeed at setting and reaching your goals is to use the S.N.A.C.K. system.

S = Small
Is this goal small enough so I can meet it in a short period of time?

N = Needed
Is this a change that I need to make for better health?

A = Achievable
Can I achieve this goal? Will I need the help of others to meet this goal? Is it a goal that I can really accomplish?

C = Can I Count it?
Is this goal written in a way that I can count and measure my progress?

K = Know-How
Do I know enough to set this health goal? Where would I find more information on this topic?

Track your progress in meeting your goals by using the goal-setting calendar on page 24.

Q. Can you think of other ways to check your progress at meeting goals? (Some ideas are listed at the bottom of the page.)

A. Some ideas: bar, line or pie graphs; write a description of how you met your goal; draw a picture of how you met your goal

Suggested Level: 3rd – 6th grade

GOAL-SETTING CALENDAR

Name ______	SUN	MON	TUE	WED	THU	FRI	SAT	MY PROGRESS:
Week 1 Dates ______ My Goal This Week: ______ ______	☐	☐	☐	☐	☐	☐	☐	☐ I met my goal! ☐ I still need to work on this: ______ ______
Week 2 Dates ______ My Goal This Week: ______ ______	☐	☐	☐	☐	☐	☐	☐	☐ I met my goal! ☐ I still need to work on this: ______ ______
Week 3 Dates ______ My Goal This Week: ______ ______	☐	☐	☐	☐	☐	☐	☐	☐ I met my goal! ☐ I still need to work on this: ______ ______
Week 4 Dates ______ My Goal This Week: ______ ______	☐	☐	☐	☐	☐	☐	☐	☐ I met my goal! ☐ I still need to work on this: ______ ______

REMEMBER TO SET S.N.A.C.K. GOALS:
Small, Needed, Achievable, Can I Count It?, Know-How

Suggested Level: 3rd – 6th grade

SAMPLE GOAL-SETTING CALENDAR

Name Hugh

	SUN	MON	TUE	WED	THU	FRI	SAT	MY PROGRESS:
Week 1 Dates 4/5–4/11 My Goal This Week: Try at least two new vegetables	X Tried jicama— YUM!	☐	X Mom put pea pods in the stir-fry	☐	☐	X At school, we had baby corn on our salad. It was OK.	☐	X I met my goal! ☐ I still need to work on this:
Week 2 Dates 4/12–4/18 My Goal This Week: Ride my bike to my friends' houses at least twice	☐	X Rode bike to Susan's	X Rode bike to Matt's (big hill!)	☐	☐	X Rode bike to Matt's again!	☐	X I met my goal! ☐ I still need to work on this:
Week 3 Dates 4/19–4/25 My Goal This Week: Eat breakfast every day this week (even if I have early band practice)	X	X Band practice - I got up earlier	X	X Slept in, but ate breakfast at school	X	X Band practice- breakfast at school	X	X I met my goal! ☐ I still need to work on this:
Week 4 Dates 4/26–5/2 My Goal This Week: Cut down on soda pop. I will drink only 3 cans instead of 7	☐ 1 can at Grandma's	X NO SODA!	☐ 1 can	☐ 1 can at Roger's house	X NO SODA!	☐ 1 can (movies)	☐ 1 can	☐ I met my goal! X I still need to work on this: I need to remember to drink water instead

REMEMBER TO SET S.N.A.C.K. GOALS:
Small, Needed, Achievable, Can I Count it?, Know-how

Suggested Level: 3rd – 6th grade

MY GOALS FOR GOOD HEALTH

Name ______________________________

This week I will work on one of the following goals for better health:

☐ Try a new vegetable or fruit.

☐ After school, I will play active games or ride my bike.

☐ Eat breakfast.

☐ Choose nutritious snacks.

☐ Drink water instead of sweetened drinks more often.

☐ Drink or eat three servings of foods from the dairy group each day.

☐ My idea for a goal: ____

____

____

"Wow, I just made a GOAL!"

Draw a picture or write a story about you and your goal for good health.

Suggested Level: K-2nd grade

BRAVO FOR BREAKFAST!

Take time to wake up your brain!

"My favorite breakfast is dinner! It's true! You can eat sandwiches, soup, pasta or even veggie pizza in the morning."

Name ______________________________

Did you know that kids who eat breakfast do better in school? That's because breakfast feeds both your body and your mind. If you are too busy to eat a healthful breakfast, try one of the following ideas:

- ☐ Get up 15 minutes earlier.
- ☐ Eat breakfast at school.
- ☐ Pack your breakfast in a bag, and eat it on the bus.
- ☐ Your ideas: ______________________________

____

Can you plan easy, nutritious breakfasts that you can fix by yourself? Aim for a breakfast that includes:

- ◆ A serving of whole grains (e.g. oatmeal, brown rice, whole grain toast, mini-bagel or waffle)
- ◆ At least one serving of fruits or vegetables
- ◆ A serving from the dairy or protein groups

My Breakfast Menus:

1. ______________________________

____

____

2. ______________________________

____

____

3. ______________________________

____

____

4. ______________________________

____

____

Suggested Level: K-6th grade

MAKE A SNACK PLAN

Name ______________________________

Snacks are an important way to keep your body fueled all day long. Think of snacks as "mini meals," made up of the same kinds of nutritious food that you eat at breakfast, lunch and dinner. Below are some examples of healthy, easy-to-fix snacks:

- Pistachios and pineapple chunks
- Peanut butter & fruit wrap using whole grain flatbread (try applesauce, sliced banana or raisins)
- Low-fat yogurt and an orange
- Whole Wheat flakes cereal with 1% or fat-free milk
- Fresh, cut-up vegetables and hummus

Now it's your turn. In the spaces below, plan four easy and nutritious snacks that you can fix by yourself. Each snack should contain at least **two** different food groups and include foods that you like.

1. ____

____

2. ____

____

3. ____

____

4. ____

____

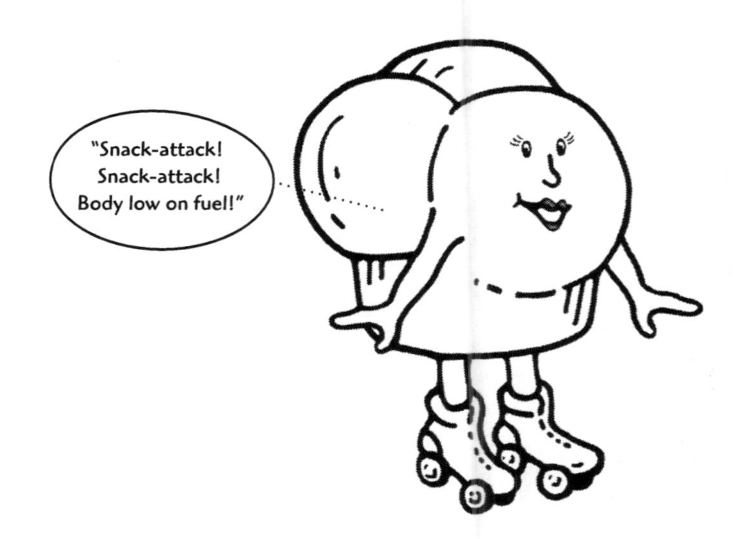

Suggested Level: K-6th grade

A ROLE-PLAYING GAME

Thinking Through Our Choices

NOTES TO EDUCATORS

Role playing in small, familiar groups is a great way for children to learn to think critically and solve nutrition-related problems. The following realistic scenarios allow children to practice making choices and explore the consequences of those choices. Stress that there are no right or wrong answers in these situations.

DIRECTIONS

Copy this page and cut out the scenarios. Divide children into small groups of two to four and give each group a different slip. Encourage children to discuss the situation and develop brief skits that demonstrate the problem and the students' solution.

Your friend thinks she is too fat, so she decides to go on a diet that she found in one of her mom's magazines. She wants you to go on the diet too. How would you handle this situation?	You always have to rush to make it to afternoon soccer practice on time. You usually grab a can of soda pop and a package of potato chips to eat on the way. The problem is your stomach often starts hurting in the middle of practice, especially if you have to run a lot. What do you think is causing your stomach aches? What changes could you make to solve this problem?
After school you always feel so hungry. When your mom's not looking, you grab a bunch of cookies and go outside to play. Later you don't feel hungry for supper. What would you do next time you're hungry after school?	Your best friend is a picky eater who rarely eats from the five food groups. You have noticed that he looks pale and tired and gets sick a lot. What could you do to help your friend?
You like it when your dad packs fruit, vegetable sticks and other healthful foods in your lunch. But the kids at school tease you about eating healthful foods, calling you "vegetable head." How would you solve this problem?	Your mom is a health food nut. She is forever bringing home strange-looking vegetables with even stranger-sounding names, things such as bok choy, kohlrabi and rutabaga! Worse yet, she expects you to eat them. You refuse, saying you will not try anything that looks or sounds strange. Is there a better way to deal with this situation?
Your friend says that a Giggles candy bar is healthful because the commercial on TV showed kids with lots of energy after they ate Giggles. He is now convinced that Giggles will give him energy too. What would you tell him?	Your big sister is pretty and popular, but all she ever eats are salads and diet soft drinks. She says most other foods are "fattening." Is she right? What would you say to her?
On school mornings you would rather sleep longer and skip breakfast. You really aren't that hungry when you first wake up anyway. But lately you have noticed that after morning recess, you have a headache, your stomach growls, and it's hard to do your work. How would you solve this problem?	Your parents went out for the evening, leaving you with a teenage babysitter. The babysitter says you can have whatever you want for dinner, even candy! What foods would you choose?

FINDING OUT MORE ABOUT THE FOOD YOU EAT

NOTES TO EDUCATORS

The activities presented in this chapter are primarily targeted to the intermediate level student. While younger students should be encouraged to begin reading *Nutrition Facts* labels, students in grades three through six can begin to take a more critical look at both food labeling and advertising.

◆ Sometimes we form opinions about food without knowing all the facts. One of the best ways to obtain a better understanding of the foods we eat is to evaluate the *Nutrition Facts* food label. After taking the quiz on page 32, students can move on to the food label exercises on pages 33 and 34.

IN THIS CHAPTER:

Label Logic
Are You a Food Fact Finder?
Potatoes
Breakfast Bars
Be an Ad-Buster
Analyzing "Frooty-Tooty Fruitsies"
A Closer Look at Saturday Morning TV
NOT SO FAST... Make a Game Plan for Eating Out

Additional *Nutrition Facts* label information and activity ideas are presented on pages 83–91 in the book *How to Teach Nutrition to Kids*.

Check out the *Nutrition Facts* Label Programs and Materials from FDA. The "Spot the Block" materials are aimed at children ages 9 to 13. To access this site, visit: http://1.usa.gov/xQZe34

◆ The "Be an Ad-Buster" activities on pages 35 and 36 help children evaluate food advertising, identify misleading claims and assess whether reading or watching food ads is a good way to learn about nutrition.

For a more thorough background on food advertising, see pages 138-144 in *How to Teach Nutrition to Kids*.

◆ Because today's families eat an increasing number of meals outside of the home, children will benefit if they learn to make healthful choices at restaurants. Many restaurant chains have nutrient information available on their Web sites, making it possible to plan a balanced menu beforehand.

For the activity on pages 37 and 38, you will need several nutrition information brochures from a variety of popular restaurants (or nutrition information from company Web sites). Before students begin this activity, review the general guidelines for meal planning included on the "Not so Fast..." worksheet on page 37 (600 to 800 calories, 20 to 25 grams of total fat and at least four food groups). This activity works well in a small-group setting.

LABEL LOGIC

Are You a Food Fact Finder?

Name ______________________________

1. Before you pour yourself a bowl of cereal, you

- **A.** make sure the box has pictures of your favorite cartoon characters.
- **B.** look at the *Nutrition Facts* label to see how much sugar, fiber and other nutrients are in one serving.
- **C.** read the front of the box to see if it brags about being healthy or nutritious.

2. You want to know if a fruit drink is really juice. You look at

- **A.** the ingredient label to see if the first ingredient is 100% fruit juice.
- **B.** the number of calories in one serving.
- **C.** the picture on the bottle to see if it looks like real fruit.

3. How would you find out if low-fat milk has as much calcium as whole milk?

- **A.** Look at the "total fat" content of each type of milk.
- **B.** Read the *Nutrition Facts* label on both types of milk and compare the "% daily value" for calcium.
- **C.** Read the *Nutrition Facts* label to see which type of milk has more calories.

4. You can't decide between "Wholelatta baloney" and "Honeygoo ham." You look at the packages to see

- **A.** which sandwich meat has the most protein and least amount of fat per serving.
- **B.** which package has more servings.
- **C.** which one looks as if it will taste better.

5. A package of your favorite peanut candy lists 250 calories per serving. You

- **A.** always share these with your friend anyway, so why worry?
- **B.** figure that one package must be one serving, so you eat the whole thing.
- **C.** look to see how many servings are in the package.

Answers: 1. B, 2. A, 3. B, 4. A, 5. C

Give yourself 5 points for each correct answer.

20–25 points: You are a pro at food fact finding!

10–15 points: Pay a little closer attention to those nutrition labels.

0–5 points: You really should try reading before eating!

"Some foods don't need ingredient labels because it is easy to see what you are getting."
Ingredients: Banana
Bananas

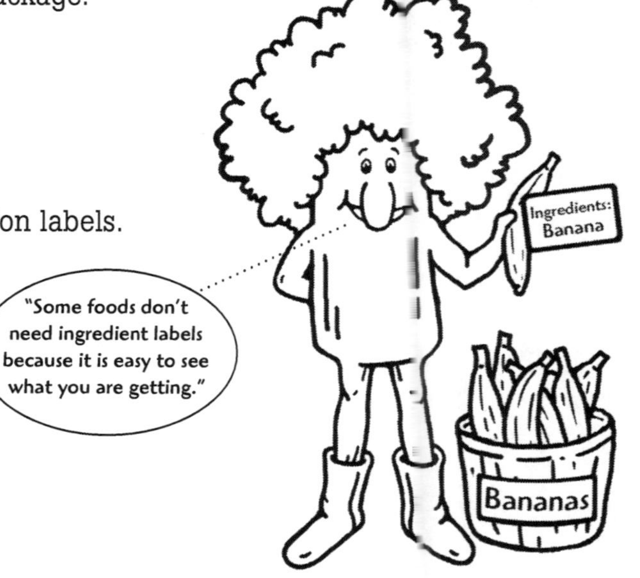

LABEL LOGIC

Potatoes

"Do you 'C' the difference here, kids?"

Name ______________________________

Fresh, unprocessed potatoes are a healthy vegetable. They are high in fiber, vitamin C and other important nutrients. This activity will help you to see how processing affects the nutritional value of potatoes.

DIRECTIONS

Use the *Nutrition Facts* food labels below to complete the information about each type of potato product. Use this information to answer the questions that follow.

Nutrition Facts	Nutrition Facts	Nutrition Facts	Nutrition Facts	Nutrition Facts
Fried Potato Crisps	Baked Potato	Hashed Brown Potatoes	French Fries (small order)	Mashed Potatoes
Serving Size 1 oz. (28g), approx 14 crisps	Serving Size 1 medium (with skin)	Serving Size 1/2 cup (78g)	Serving Size 15 fries (74g)	Serving Size 1/2 cup (105g)
Amount Per Serving	Amount Per Serving	Amount Per Serving	Amount Per Serving	Amount Per Serving
Calories 158 Calories from Fat 99	Calories 150 Calories from Fat 0	Calories 163 Calories from Fat 99	Calories 250 Calories from Fat 120	Calories 111 Calories from Fat 36
% Daily Value*	% Daily Value*	% Daily Value*	% Daily Value*	% Daily Value*
Total Fat 11g 17%	Total Fat 0g 0%	Total Fat 11g 17%	Total Fat 13g 20%	Total Fat 4g 6%
Saturated Fat 3g 15%	Saturated Fat 0g 0%	Saturated Fat 4g 20%	Saturated Fat 2.5g 13%	Saturated Fat 1g 5%
Trans Fat 0g	Trans Fat 0g	Trans Fat 4g	Trans Fat 3.5g	Trans Fat 0g
Cholesterol 0 mg 0%	Cholesterol 0 mg 0%	Cholesterol 0 mg 0%	Cholesterol 0 mg 0%	Cholesterol 13 mg 4%
Sodium 186 mg 8%	Sodium 11 mg <1%	Sodium 19 mg 1%	Sodium 140 mg 6%	Sodium 309 mg 13%
Total Carbohydrate 14g 5%	Total Carbohydrate 35g 12%	Total Carbohydrate 17g 6%	Total Carbohydrate 30g 10%	Total Carbohydrate 18g 6%
Dietary Fiber 1g 4%	Dietary Fiber 3g 12%	Dietary Fiber 0g 0%	Dietary Fiber 3g 12%	Dietary Fiber 1g 4%
Sugars 0g	Sugars 2g	Sugars 0g	Sugars 0g	Sugars 4g
Protein 2g	Protein 3g	Protein 2g	Protein 2g	Protein 2g
Vitamin A 0% Vitamin C 6%	Vitamin A 0% Vitamin C 30%	Vitamin A 0% Vitamin C 8%	Vitamin A 0% Vitamin C 6%	Vitamin A 4% Vitamin C 10%
Calcium 0% Iron 0%	Calcium 1% Iron 10%	Calcium 0% Iron 4%	Calcium 2% Iron 4%	Calcium 3% Iron 2%
*Percent Daily Values are based on a 2,000-calorie diet.	*Percent Daily Values are based on a 2,000-calorie diet.	*Percent Daily Values are based on a 2,000-calorie diet.	*Percent Daily Values are based on a 2,000-calorie diet.	*Percent Daily Values are based on a 2,000-calorie diet.

Grams of total fat in one serving ______	Grams of total fat in one serving ______	Grams of total fat in one serving ______	Grams of total fat in one serving ______	Grams of total fat in one serving ______
Vitamin C ______ (% Daily Value)	Vitamin C ______ (% Daily Value)	Vitamin C ______ (% Daily Value)	Vitamin C ______ (% Daily Value)	Vitamin C ______ (% Daily Value)

1. Compare the fat content of the different types of potato products. Rank them from lowest to highest:
   ____
   ____

2. Compare the vitamin C content of the different types of potato products. Rank them from lowest to highest: ____
   ____

3. In general, what happens to the vitamin C in a potato as it is processed into other products?
   ____
   ____

4. Which of the potato choices do you think is the most nutritious? Explain how you came up with this answer. ____
   ____

Suggested Level: 3rd - 6th grade

LABEL LOGIC

Breakfast Bars

Name ______________________________

Are breakfast bars a good way to start the day? Many breakfast bars that appear to be healthy are actually loaded with sugar and fat and fall short on nutrients such as protein and fiber. See if you can tell which of the bars below is the most nutritious choice.

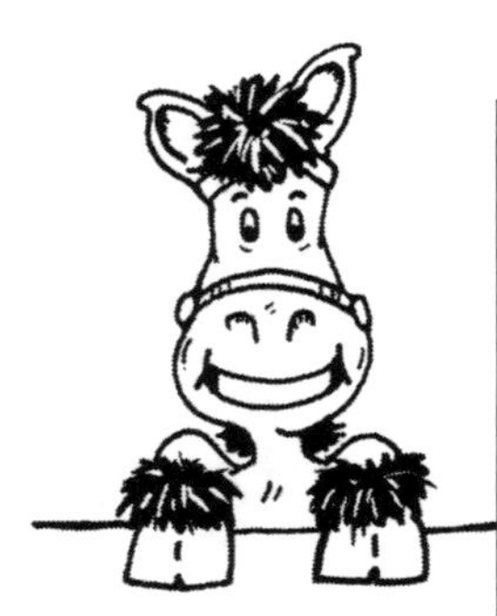

Giddyup & Go Bars

Nutrition Facts	
Serving Size 1 bar (40g)	
Servings per container 5	
Amount Per Serving	
Calories 160	Calories from Fat 30
	% Daily Value*
Total Fat 3g	**5%**
Saturated Fat 0.5g	**3%**
Trans fat 0g	
Cholesterol 0 mg	**0%**
Sodium 70 mg	**3%**
Total Carbohydrate 29g	**10%**
Dietary Fiber 4g	**11%**
Sugars 8g	
Protein 4g	
Vitamin A 0%	Vitamin C 0%
Calcium 10%	Iron 8%

*Percent Daily Values are based on a 2,000-calorie diet.

Wake-Up Mighty Munch Bars

Nutrition Facts	
Serving Size 1 bar (39g)	
Servings per container 8	
Amount Per Serving	
Calories 150	Calories from Fat 36
	% Daily Value*
Total Fat 4g	**6%**
Saturated Fat 1g	**5%**
Trans fat 0g	
Cholesterol 0 mg	**0%**
Sodium 75 mg	**3%**
Total Carbohydrate 28g	**9%**
Dietary Fiber 1g	**4%**
Sugars 20g	
Protein 1g	
Vitamin A 0%	Vitamin C 0%
Calcium 2%	Iron 4%

*Percent Daily Values are based on a 2,000-calorie diet.

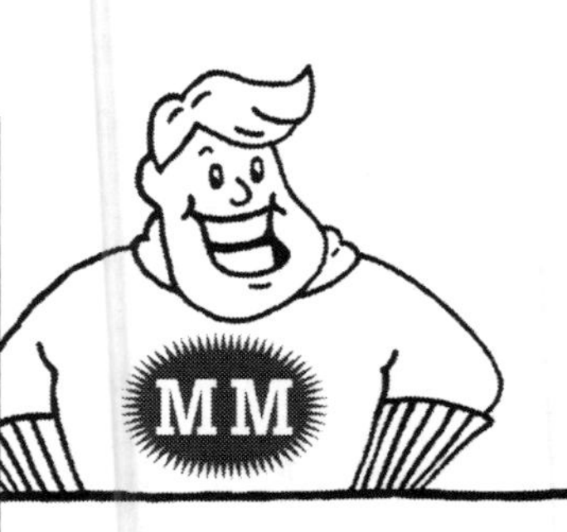

1. Which bar has the most sugar?______________________________

2. Which bar is highest in fat?______________________________

3. Name the bar with the most:

Fiber ______________________ Protein ______________________

Iron ______________________ Calcium ______________________

4. Which bar is the best nutritional choice?______________________________

"Fiber is good stuff! It works like a broom to sweep out your digestive system."

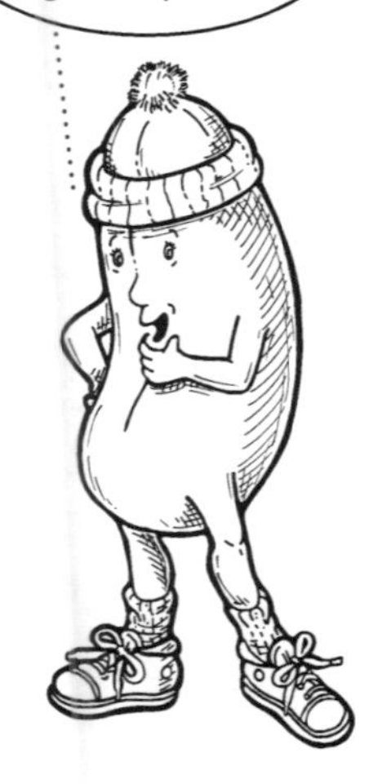

Answer: Giddyup & Go Bars have the least amount of sugar and fat and the most protein, fiber, iron and calcium. They are definitely the best choice.

Suggested Level: 3rd - 6th grade

BE AN AD-BUSTER

Analyzing "Frooty-Tooty Fruitsies"

Name ______________________________

Did you know that food advertising can sometimes make a food sound more nutritious than it really is? You need to take a close look at the food label to determine if the food lives up to the advertising claims.

DIRECTIONS

Read the advertisement for "Frooty-Tooty Fruitsies." (It's made up, by the way.) Next, study the ***Nutrition Facts*** label for this product and answer the questions below.

WHAT THE ADVERTISEMENT SAYS:

Frooty-Tooty Fruitsies give your body a high-energy boost. They are bursting with FRUIT flavor and wholesome goodness. Frooty-Tooty Fruitsies make a Fruity-licious Nutritious Treat!!

Nutrition Facts
Frooty-Tooty Fruitsies
Serving Size 15 pieces
Servings Per Container 1

Amount Per Serving	
Calories 120	Calories from Fat 0
	% Daily Value*
Total Fat 0g	0%
Saturated Fat 0g	0%
Trans Fat 0g	
Cholesterol 0 mg	0%
Sodium 45 mg	2%
Total Carbohydrate 29g	10%
Dietary Fiber 0g	0%
Sugars 23g	
Protein 1g	
Vitamin A 0%	Vitamin C 0%
Calcium 0%	Iron 0%

*Percent Daily Values are based on a 2,000-calorie diet.

WHAT THE LABEL SHOWS:

Ingredients: High-fructose corn syrup, sugar, gelatin, fruit juice concentrate, artificial flavorings, artificial colorings.

1. The ingredients listed on a food label are listed from most to least. Look at the ingredient label for **Frooty-Tooty Fruitsies.** How many of the first three ingredients are forms of sugar? Are any of the ingredients listed a source of real fruit? ______________________________

____

2. Real fruit and 100% fruit juices tend to contribute vitamins A and C to the diet. Are **Frooty-Tooty Fruitsies** a good source of either of these vitamins? ______________________________

____

3. Do you think that **Frooty-Tooty Fruitsies** are a "Fruity-licious Nutritious" treat? Why or why not?

____

____

4. Can you think of an example of a food advertisement that you have seen that makes misleading claims about nutrition? Describe it below.

____

____

Suggested Level: 3rd - 6th grade

BE AN AD-BUSTER
A Closer Look at Saturday Morning TV

Name ______________________________

DIRECTIONS

To complete this activity, you will watch at least one hour of Saturday morning programming on a commercial television network, such as ABC, CBS, NBC, Fox or Nickelodeon. Once you decide on the channel, do not switch networks until you have finished this assignment.

NETWORK WATCHED ____________________ WHAT TIME DID YOU START WATCHING? ______________

DATE WATCHED ________________________ WHAT TIME DID YOU STOP WATCHING? ______________

Every time you see a food commercial, make a tally mark beside the category below that best describes the food advertised.

____________ Candy
____________ Soft drinks
____________ Sweetened beverages (not 100% fruit juice)
____________ Sweetened cereal
____________ Corn chips, potato chips or other fried snacks
____________ Cakes, cookies or pastries
____________ Sweetened fruit snacks
____________ Other sweetened foods

FOOD GROUPS

____________ Grains (breads, low-sugar cereals, waffles, pasta, rice)
____________ Fruits (fresh, frozen or canned; 100% fruit juices)
____________ Vegetables (fresh, frozen or canned; vegetable juices)
____________ Protein (meat, fish, chicken, beans, eggs, peanut butter)
____________ Dairy (milk, cheese, yogurt)

OTHERS

____________ Combination Meals (examples: pizza, children's frozen dinners)
____________ Fast-Food Restaurants
____________ Public Service Announcements promoting good nutrition
____________ ____
____________ ____

How many total food advertisements did you see during the time you watched? ______________

How many of these were for foods that you consider nutritious? ______________

How many of these were for foods that are not the most nutritious? ______________

Do you think there should be more advertisements for healthful foods on television? Why or why not?

____

NOT SO FAST... Make a Game Plan for Eating Out

Name ______________________________

Planning ahead is the key to choosing more balanced meals when eating at restaurants. The nutrition advice in the box below will help you plan a more balanced meal. Using the planning sheet on page 38, see if you can plan restaurant meals that meet the following calorie, fat and food group guidelines.

MENU PLANNING GUIDELINES (per meal)

- ◆ 600-800 total calories for one meal
- ◆ 20-25 grams of fat for one meal
- ◆ At least four different food groups in each meal

EXAMPLE

RESTAURANT Burrito Hut

Food Item	Calories	Fat Grams	Food Groups
Chicken Burrito with cheese	360	12	Protein, Grains, Dairy
Salsa (3 ounces)	27	0	Vegetables
Mexican Rice (1/2 cup)	110	3	Grains
Cinnamon Chips (1 ounce)	139	6	Grains (& 1 serving of "Extras")
Bottled Water	0	0	None
Totals:	636	21	4 different food groups

See page 38 for copy-ready restaurant planning sheets.

"Pasta, sandwiches, fresh fruit, salads and milk are fast foods that you can find or make at home!"

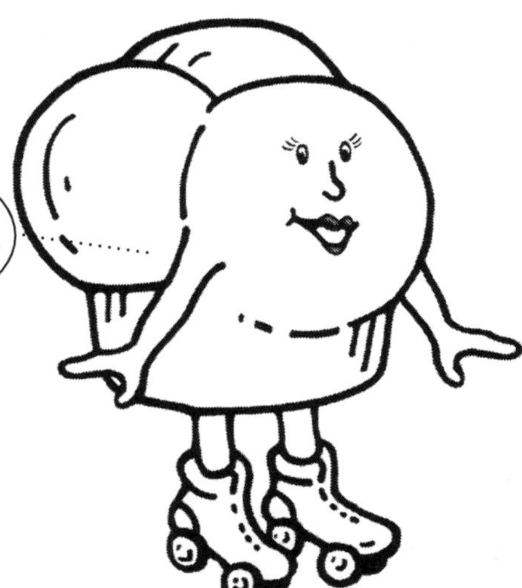

Suggested Level: 3rd - 6th grade

RESTAURANT ______________________

Food Item	Calories	Fat Grams	Food Groups
Totals:			

RESTAURANT ______________________

Food Item	Calories	Fat Grams	Food Groups
Totals:			

RESTAURANT ______________________

Food Item	Calories	Fat Grams	Food Groups
Totals:			

COOKING UP SOME FUN

NOTES TO EDUCATORS

Nutrition education takes on a whole new life when combined with cooking projects. Learning to cook gives children a boost in confidence, exposure to new and healthy foods and inspiration to continue cooking at home.

IN THIS CHAPTER:

Wacky Snacks:
- Tortizza
- Burrato
- Yobanola
- My Wacky Snacks

Make Your Own Recipes:
- Egg-Xactly Right Eggs
- Fuel-Up Trail Mix
- Perfectly Personal Pizza
- Soup Like You Like it
- Stir-Fry Surprise

Recipe Review

The activities on the following pages allow children to creatively experiment within a basic framework of tried-and-true recipes. Most of the recipes in this chapter can be prepared by kids of all ages. Younger children will need closer supervision, however.

Before you begin, send a letter home to parents explaining that their children will be participating in cooking projects that enhance the curriculum. *Be sure to elicit information about food allergies or intolerances or any specific medical conditions that prohibit children from eating certain foods.* Include permission slips for parents to sign and return.

When cooking with children, it is always important to stress the importance of safety and sanitation when handling food. Instruct children to always wash their hands before food preparation and whenever they use the restroom or touch their hair, nose or neighbor. Closely supervise children's use of knives, equipment, microwaves, ovens and other cooking surfaces. The appendix on pages 203–206 in *How to Teach Nutrition to Kids* offers specific guidance for keeping cooking projects safe and sanitary.

Creative cooking projects also make great homework assignments. Encourage students to try one of the recipes suggested here or create one of their own. The *Recipe Review* form on page 47 should be completed for each recipe that you assign.

NOTE: Look for other recipes on the bottom of the food group puzzle sheets in Chapter 6.

WACKY SNACKS

"A wacky snack is a mixture of foods that tastes delicious and has a funny name."

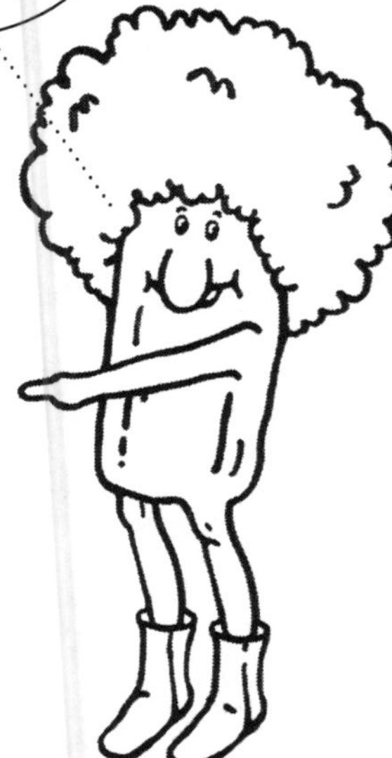

Tortilla + Pizza = TORTIZZA!

INGREDIENTS

1 10" whole-wheat flour tortilla

2 T. prepared pizza or pasta sauce

1/4 cup grated part-skim mozzarella cheese

1/4 cup chopped vegetables of your choice
(examples include peppers, mushrooms, onions and broccoli florets)

DIRECTIONS

Spread sauce evenly over tortilla. Add cheese and vegetables and roll up the tortilla. Microwave on high for 1 minute. *Makes 1 serving*

Burrito + Potato = BURRATO!

INGREDIENTS

1 medium potato

1-2 T. salsa

2 T. refried beans (or refried black beans)

2 T. grated sharp cheddar cheese

DIRECTIONS

Wash and scrub potato. Using a sharp knife, carefully poke the potato (this allows the steam to escape during cooking). Microwave on high for 4-6 minutes. After the potato has cooled, cut in half, press down to flatten, and spread remaining ingredients evenly between the two potato halves. Microwave on high for 1 minute. Optional: Serve with low-fat sour cream or plain Greek yogurt, shredded lettuce, cilantro and avocado chunks.
Makes 1 serving

"Substitute berries for the banana and you have a YOBERROLA."

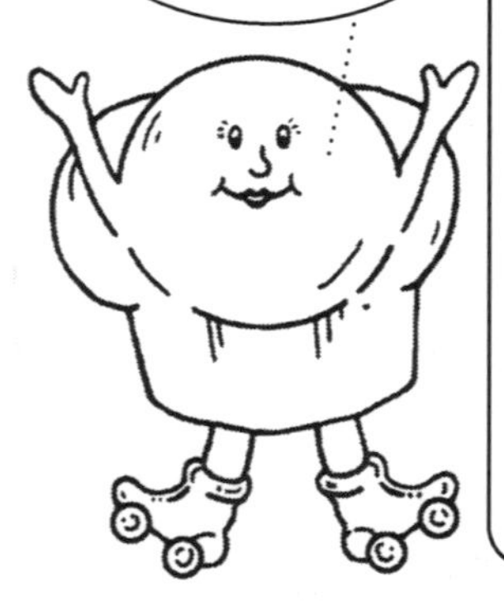

Yogurt + Banana + Granola = YOBANOLA!

INGREDIENTS

1 6-8 oz. carton low-fat or fat-free vanilla yogurt

1 banana

1/4 cup low-fat granola cereal

DIRECTIONS

Peel and slice banana. Divide between two cereal-sized bowls. Top the bananas with the yogurt (one-half carton per bowl). Sprinkle granola on top of each bowl.
Makes 2 servings (share with a friend!)

MY WACKY SNACKS

How do you make a wacky snack? By mixing two or more foods together, you get a delicious snack with a funny name.

"Why did the peas and carrots fly away?"

"Because when they were mixed, they turned into parrots!"

____________'s WACKY SNACK RECIPE

NAME

____________ + ____________ + ____________ = ____________

INGREDIENTS:

____

____

____

____

DIRECTIONS:

____

____

____

____

____________'s WACKY SNACK RECIPE

NAME

____________ + ____________ + ____________ = ____________

INGREDIENTS:

____

____

____

____

DIRECTIONS:

____

____

____

____

Suggested Level: 1st - 6th grade

MAKE YOUR OWN RECIPE
Egg-Xactly Right Eggs

Name ______________________________

This recipe is a fool-proof way for the beginning cook to learn to make fluffy scrambled eggs.

Equipment needed: mixing bowl, measuring cup, microweavable dish with lid, wire whisk or fork

BASIC RECIPE

INGREDIENTS

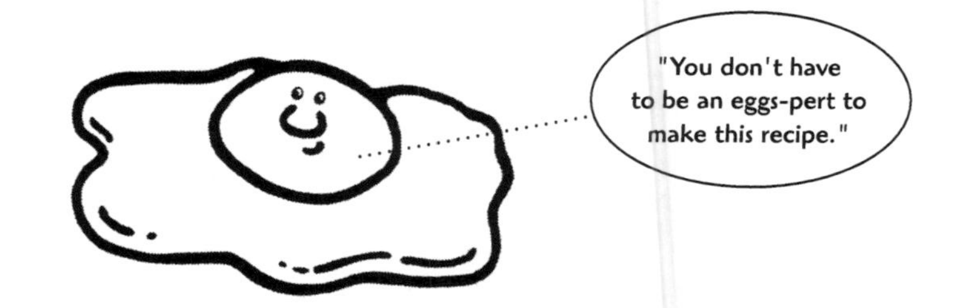

4 medium eggs
1/4 cup fat-free or 1% milk
non stick spray
salt & pepper to taste

DIRECTIONS

Spray the microwaveable dish with non stick spray. Crack the eggs in the mixing bowl, add milk and stir well with wire whisk or fork. Pour into microwaveable dish, cover and microwave on high for 3–4 minutes. Carefully remove eggs from the microwave using pot holders. Remove the lid and use a spoon to break the eggs into bite-sized pieces. Add a small amount of salt and pepper or try one of the variations below. Be creative!
Makes 2–3 servings

VARIATIONS

Eggs Olé—After you remove eggs from the microwave, top with 2 tablespoons of salsa, 5 sliced black olives, and 2 tablespoons of grated cheddar cheese. Replace lid and let eggs sit for 1–2 more minutes.

Greek Eggs – Add 1/2 teaspoon of dried oregano to the basic recipe prior to cooking. After you remove eggs from the microwave, top with 2 tablespoons of fresh, chopped tomato and 2–3 tablespoons of crumbled feta cheese. Replace lid and let eggs sit for 1–2 more minutes.

Pita Pocket Veggie Breakfast – Stuff a pita pocket with scrambled eggs, 2 tablespoons of grated mozzarella or jack cheese, and chopped vegetables of your choice such as onions, green pepper, asparagus chunks, baby spinach or sun-dried tomatoes.

My Own Egg-Xactly Right Variations

____

____

____

____

MAKE YOUR OWN RECIPE

Fuel-Up Trail Mix

Name ______________________________

Fuel-Up Trail Mix makes a great snack to put in your backpack, your gym bag or the car. It is delicious and easy to make!

Equipment needed: measuring cups and spoons, medium-sized bowl, plastic bags or airtight plastic containers

DIRECTIONS

1. Using a 1/4 cup measuring cup, mix equal amounts of some or all of the following ingredients in a bowl:
   - ☐ Low-fat granola cereal
   - ☐ Quick-cooking oatmeal
   - ☐ Low-sugar breakfast cereal
   - ☐ Small pretzel sticks or twists
   - ☐ Shelled sunflower seeds
   - ☐ Peanuts
   - ☐ Almonds
   - ☐ Raisins
   - ☐ Dried cranberries
   - ☐ Dried apple rings
   - ☐ Dried apricots
   - ☐ Dried blueberries

   Other ingredients:
   - ☐ ______________________________
   - ☐ ______________________________
2. Mix in 1–2 teaspoons of **ONE** of the following:
   - ☐ Chocolate chips
   - ☐ Candy coated peanuts
   - ☐ Other small candies
3. Store in plastic bags or airtight plastic containers.

My Very Own, Very Favorite Fuel-Up Trail Mix Recipe

____

____

____

____

Suggested Level: 1st - 6th grade

MAKE YOUR OWN RECIPE

Perfectly Personal Pizza

"With practice, you can make this recipe quicker than the pizza delivery guy can find your house!"

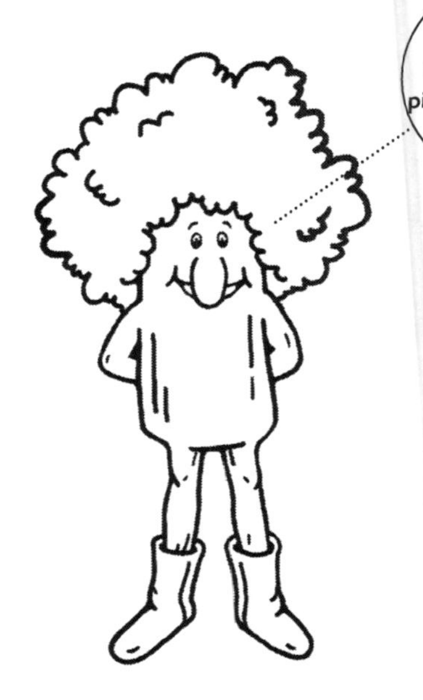

Name ______________________________

Equipment needed: 15–16" pizza pan, measuring cups and spoons, mixing bowl, cutting board and knife

CRUST RECIPE

INGREDIENTS

1 package active dry yeast
1 cup warm tap water
1 teaspoon sugar
1/2 teaspoon salt
2 tablespoons canola oil
2-1/2 cups whole-wheat flour
non stick spray

DIRECTIONS

Preheat oven to 400° F. Lightly spray pizza pan with non stick spray. Dissolve yeast in warm water. Stir in remaining ingredients, and mix until you can form into a ball of dough. Set aside for five minutes. Next, spread dough out on pizza pan until it covers the entire pan. (HINT: The dough will be easier to work with if you dip your fingers in flour.) Bake in preheated oven for 10 minutes.

TOPPING IT OFF

INGREDIENTS

1/2 to 3/4 cup prepared pizza sauce
8 ounces part-skim mozzarella cheese
Toppings of your choice

DIRECTIONS

1. Once your crust is pre-baked, spread the pizza sauce evenly over the crust.
2. Sprinkle 8 ounces of grated part-skim mozzarella cheese over the sauce.
3. Add one or more of the following toppings (you decide how much):
   - ☐ Pepper rings (red, green, yellow or orange)
   - ☐ Sliced mushrooms
   - ☐ Sliced olives
   - ☐ Broccoli florets
   - ☐ Tomato slices
   - ☐ Onions, chopped or sliced
   - ☐ Canadian bacon
   - ☐ Lean ham, thinly sliced
   - ☐ Browned meat crumbles (lean ground beef or ground turkey)
4. Bake at 400° for 10 more minutes or until cheese is slightly browned. *Makes 8 servings.*

MAKE YOUR OWN RECIPE

Soup Like You Like It

Name ______________________________

Equipment Needed: large cooking pot, measuring cups and spoons, can opener

Ingredients: Pick **ONE** choice in each category for this recipe:

1. Broth* (2 cups): ☐ Vegetable ☐ Chicken ☐ Beef

2. Juice* (3 cups): ☐ Vegetable juice ☐ Tomato juice

3. Vegetables:
- ☐ 1 pound bag of frozen peas, corn, green beans or various mixed vegetable combinations
- ☐ 3–4 cups fresh, cut-up vegetables such as carrots, potatoes, zucchini or cabbage
- ☐ Combination of frozen and fresh vegetables (3–4 cups total)

4. Protein:
- ☐ 1 can (approximately 16 ounces) kidney, pinto, navy or black beans, drained*
- ☐ 2 cups of lean meat, such as cut-up turkey or ham, or cooked roast beef

5. Pasta:
- ☐ 1 cup of your favorite shaped whole grain pasta such as penne, rotini or bowties

6. All of the following:
- ☐ 1/2 teaspoon garlic powder
- ☐ 1 teaspoon Italian seasoning
- ☐ 1/2 teaspoon pepper
- ☐ 1 cup water

"To make this meal complete, just add whole-grain bread or crackers, fresh fruit and grated Parmesan cheese."

**May substitute low-sodium varieties of these ingredients*

DIRECTIONS

In large cooking pot, combine broth, juice, vegetables, protein ingredient, water, garlic, Italian seasoning and pepper. Cook on medium heat until soup boils. Add pasta and cook for 15–20 minutes, until pasta is tender.
Makes 8–10 servings

Notes on My Favorite Ingredients for This Recipe

____

____

____

____

MAKE YOUR OWN RECIPE

Stir-Fry Surprise

Name ______________________________

Equipment Needed: measuring cups and spoons, small bowl, cutting board and knife, grater, large non stick skillet or wok

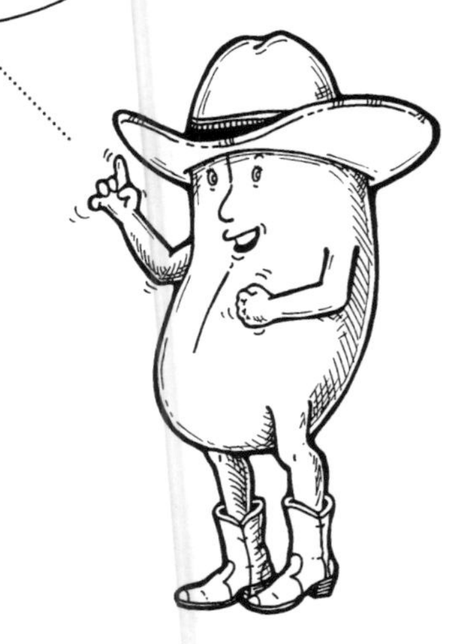

"To make this a complete one-dish meal, add chunks of tofu, cooked chicken, shrimp or lean beef along with the veggies at step 4."

INGREDIENTS FOR STIR-FRY SAUCE

1/4 cup light soy sauce
1/4 cup pineapple juice
1/4 cup rice vinegar
2 tablespoons honey
1/4 teaspoon garlic powder
1 teaspoon ground ginger
1 T. cornstarch

DIRECTIONS

1. Mix together soy sauce, pineapple juice, rice vinegar, honey, garlic powder, ground ginger and cornstarch. Set aside.

2. Choose some or all of the following vegetables (to equal about 6 cups total):

- ☐ Peppers (red, green, yellow or orange)
- ☐ Green onions
- ☐ Grated carrots
- ☐ Pea pods
- ☐ Broccoli
- ☐ Cauliflower
- ☐ Mushrooms
- ☐ Eggplant
- ☐ Baby corn
- ☐ Asparagus
- ☐ Bok choy
- ☐ Other veggies ________________

3. Using a cutting board and sharp knife, cut up vegetables into bite-sized pieces. Grate carrots.

4. Heat 2–3 tablespoons canola or olive oil in a large skillet or wok on medium-high heat. Add vegetables and stir 3–5 minutes or until tender. Pour stir-fry sauce over vegetables and cook 1–2 minutes longer.

5. Serve over brown rice, quinoa, whole wheat couscous, noodles, pasta or alone as a side dish. Or try wrapping up the veggies in a whole corn tortilla.

Makes 4 servings

RECIPE REVIEW

Name ______________________________

"This is homework the dog really could eat!"

DIRECTIONS

Ask your teacher for copies of the *Wacky Snacks* or *Make Your Own Recipe* sheets. Pick a recipe that you would like to try or use a recipe idea of your own. When you are finished, be sure to complete this worksheet.

GOOD COOK REMINDERS!

Every time I cook, I need to remember to

1. ask permission.
2. wash my hands and work area.
3. gather all of the ingredients.
4. gather all of the equipment.
5. prepare the recipe.
6. clean up my work area.
7. fill out this work sheet.

The recipe I tried at home was:

This is how I made this recipe:

This is how it looked:

This is how it tasted:

Changes to try the next time I make this recipe:

______________________________ tasted my recipe.

Adult Signature

Adult comments are welcome: ______________________________

Suggested Level: 1st - 6th grade

GROWING FUN

NOTES TO EDUCATORS

Besides the many opportunities for active learning, gardening entices kids to prepare and eat a wider variety of fruits, vegetables, herbs, legumes and grains.

Gardening with children provides a myriad of teachable moments and learning opportunities. Science, ecology and nutrition concepts are all a logical extension of the garden. Kids can also gain skills in language arts, math, art and social studies. Encourage children to write, graph and draw pictures about the garden and its changes throughout the season. Check out books on how other cultures grow and use food. Share the garden harvest with food banks or homeless shelters in the community.

IN THIS CHAPTER:

- Get Started in the Garden (Checklist)
- Keep a Garden Journal
- Plant a Theme Garden
- Grow an Indoor Herb Garden
- Discover Food Where You Live

This chapter is an introduction to the gardening experience. The resources below and those listed throughout this section provide detailed and comprehensive information on how to become a "growing classroom."

Suggested Resources:

Agriculture in the Classroom — *www.agclassroom.org*
California Ag in the Classroom — *www.cfaitc.org*
California School Garden Network — *www.csgn.org*
Garden ABCs — *www.gardenabcs.com*
Kids Gardening — *www.kidsgardening.org*
Life Lab — *www.lifelab.org*
People's Garden from USDA — *www.usda.gov/peoplesgarden*
Team Nutrition School Garden Site — *healthymeals.nal.usda.gov/hsmrs/garden/*
The Edible Schoolyard Project — *www.edibleschoolyard.org*

Books:

Bucklin-Sporer, A. & Pringle, R. (2010). *How to Grow a School Garden.* Portland, OR: Timber Press.

Lovejoy, S. (1999). *Roots, shoots, buckets & boots: gardening together with children.* New York: Workman Pub.

Patten, E. & Lyons, K. (2003). *Healthy foods from healthy soils: a hands-on resource for educators.* Gardner, Me: Tilbury House Publishers.

GET STARTED IN THE GARDEN

Name_______________________________

Growing vegetables from seeds is both fun and tasty. Review the checklist below to make sure you have everything you need to get started. Be sure to ask an adult for help in planning and planting your garden.

THINGS YOU WILL NEED

☐ **Good Soil**

Garden soil should be dark brown and feel loose in your hands. It is best to start with containers or garden beds that you can fill with an organic compost-rich soil.

☐ **Light**

Be sure to find a sunny location for your plants to grow. Inside, a south-facing window is best for starting or growing plants.

☐ **Water**

☐ **Natural Fertilizer**

Fertilizers add nitrogen, potassium and phosphorous to your soil. Many garden centers and catalogs sell organic fertilizers that are suitable for growing fruits, vegetables and herbs.

☐ **Garden Tools**

You will need tools such as a shovel, rake, hoe, watering can and gloves. Buckets and wheelbarrows also come in handy for hauling dirt and compost around the garden.
Other tools I need for my garden: ____

☐ **Seeds**

Of course, you need seeds to start your vegetable garden. You can get many different types of seeds from local garden centers, web sites and catalogs. Always follow the directions on the seed packet. The packet tells you where, when and how to plant the seeds, instructions for plant care and many other details about growing and harvesting.

☐ **A Gardening Plan**

Before you get started, come up with a plan for your garden. Decide what you will grow, when and where you will plant your garden and who will help you get the things you need. It is helpful to draw a diagram or map of your garden.

YOU ALSO NEED TO KNOW

"It's no surprise that broccoli is a cool vegetable!"

☐ **Your growing zone**

There are 11 growing zones in the United States. You can find your zone by visiting ***www.garden.org/zipzone*** and entering your ZIP code. Knowing and understanding your zone will help you to decide when to plant different kinds of vegetables.

Cool-weather vegetables can be planted in early spring, after there is little danger of frost. Examples include lettuce, spinach, greens, radishes, broccoli and carrots.

Hot-weather vegetables can be planted outdoors when the overnight temperatures are 50 degrees or warmer. To get a head start, plant hot-weather crops such as tomatoes, peppers, eggplant and squash indoors in small pots and transfer them outdoors when it warms up.

KEEP A GARDEN JOURNAL

Name ______________________________

Date ______________________________

Weather ______________________________

Describe what you did today in the garden (planning, tilling, planting, weeding, watering, harvesting, observing, relaxing, etc.) ______________________________

____

____

____

____

What changes did you see since your last visit? ______________________________

____

____

____

____

____

Things I should do to keep my garden growing: ______________________________

____

____

____

____

____

Pictures, stories or poems about my garden:

Suggested Level: 1st - 6th grade

PLANT A THEME GARDEN

Name______________________________

A fun way to garden is to dream up a special theme, make a plan and plant your special garden. Here are some ideas to get you started.

☐ **A growing salad bowl**
It's easy to grow leaf lettuce, romaine lettuce, spinach and other salad greens. Most lettuce varieties prefer weather that is on the cool side so spring and fall are normally the best time to grow salad greens. Plant seeds directly into your outside garden plot.

☐ **Plant a pizza**
A pizza garden has most of the ingredients to top your pizza. Tomatoes, peppers, onions, garlic and herbs such as oregano and basil can be grown in your pizza plot. Just add the crust and cheese to make it complete.

☐ **Salsa garden**
Plant tomatoes, onions, garlic, spicy peppers and cilantro in your salsa garden.

☐ **Root garden**
Devote one garden bed to growing root vegetables. In addition to familiar root veggies such as radishes and carrots, try growing turnips, parsnips, ginger and tubers such as potatoes and sweet potatoes.

☐ **Ethnic theme**
Grow bok choy to use in Chinese soup, red beets to make Russian borscht (a soup), jalapeños to spice up Mexican food, eggplants and roma tomatoes for Italian fare or other ethnic foods that you are interested in growing.

My ideas for a theme garden: ____

____

____

____

____

GROW AN INDOOR HERB GARDEN

Name_______________________________

You can grow an herb garden indoors, even in the chilly winter months. As long as you have a source of light, you can grow delicious herbs that add flavor and fun to your favorite foods.

YOU WILL NEED

small peat pots or peat pellets, soilless planting mix,* 4" pots (for transplanting), herb seeds such as basil, parsley, chives, cilantro, dill, chamomile, cress and fennel.

**You can find soilless planting mix at a garden center. You can also make your own planting mix by combining 1/3 part sand, 1/3 part peat moss and 1/3 part organic potting soil. If you use peat pellets, you will not need the soilless mix until you transplant into the larger container.*

DIRECTIONS

1. Fill the peat pots with the soilless planting mix. If you are using peat pellets, place in a shallow bowl or container and add warm water to hydrate the pellets. The pellets will grow to a height of about 2".
2. Follow the directions on the seed packages and plant 3–4 seeds in each peat pot or pellet.
3. Place the pots inside a shallow bowl or other shallow container and set in a sunny window (south-facing is the best). Indoor grow lights will also work if you don't have a sunny window.
4. Water the pots from the bottom only. Do this by adding water to the shallow bowl or container. Add a little water at a time, until it is all soaked up and the pots are damp.
5. Check on your pots each day. Water as needed but don't soak the pots.
6. After a week or two, you will see sprouts in your pot. When they begin to grow, thin the plants to one per pot.
7. Once your plant is 2–3 inches tall, you can put it in a larger pot filled with soilless planting mixture. Fill the larger pot 2/3 full and place the entire peat pot or pellet inside the pot. Fill in the edges with the planting mix.
8. Continue to water and keep in a sunny place.
9. Use the leaves from your favorite herbs to flavor your food. (Be sure to wash the leaves well before tasting.)

My notes on growing and tasting herbs: ____

____

____

____

____

Suggested Level: 3rd - 6th grade

DISCOVER FOOD WHERE YOU LIVE

Name_____________________________

Eating closer to home

While much of the food you eat comes from places far away (sometimes thousands of miles), it is important to also include foods that are grown nearby. Here are some reasons to eat more locally:

- Fruits and vegetables retain more of their nutrients when they are eaten soon after harvest.
- Fresh food tastes better.
- Food is cheaper if it doesn't have to travel hundreds or even thousands of miles.
- Can you think of other reasons to eat locally produced foods?______________________________

  ____

  ____

Think outside the store

Some grocery markets feature foods that are grown, caught or made close by. In many places, you can also buy food directly from the farmer or rancher who produced it.

- **Farm direct stores** are stores or stands found at local farms that sell food directly to customers.
- A **farmers' market** is a place where many farmers and ranchers get together and set up stands where you can buy local food.
- Of course, you can also grow some of your own food in a **home garden.**

ACTIVITIES

☐ Be a food geographer!

The next time you visit the grocery store, take some time to check out where your food was made, caught or grown. For fresh fruits, read those little stickers to see which state or country the fruit came from. For packaged and processed foods, check the label to see where the food was grown or processed. Count how many places your food came from. Plot your results on a world map.

☐ Design a "*MyPlate* where I live"

Research the foods that are grown in your state or region. Using the blank *MyPlate* on page 11, fill in all of the agricultural products that you have identified in the correct food group spaces. To learn more about what is grown in your state or nearby states, visit *http://www.agclassroom.org/kids/ag_facts.htm* and click on the state.

☐ Locate local food

Find out where the farm direct stores and farmers' markets are in your area by visiting *www.localharvest.org* and entering your ZIP code.

PUZZLES, ACTIVITIES & MORE RECIPES

NOTES TO EDUCATORS

Use the activity sheets in this chapter to introduce a nutrition unit or reinforce nutrition concepts. Provide as handouts in the cafeteria, at health fairs or during wellness week. The sheets also work well as homework assignments that children can share with family members. Encourage children to try the simple recipes included on the activity sheets.

IN THIS CHAPTER:

- Use Your Brain to Find Whole Grains
- Veggie Plant Parts
- Fruit: Nature's Sweet Treats
- The Protein Scene
- A M-O-O-O-O-VING Story About Dairy
- A Month of Fitness & Fun! Calendar
- It's Hugh-Man (and the Foodettes) Puppet Page

PUZZLE SOLUTIONS

USE YOUR BRAIN TO FIND WHOLE GRAINS

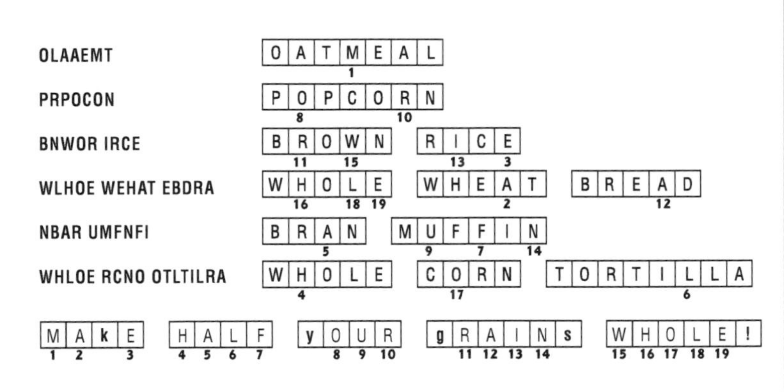

VEGGIE PLANT PARTS

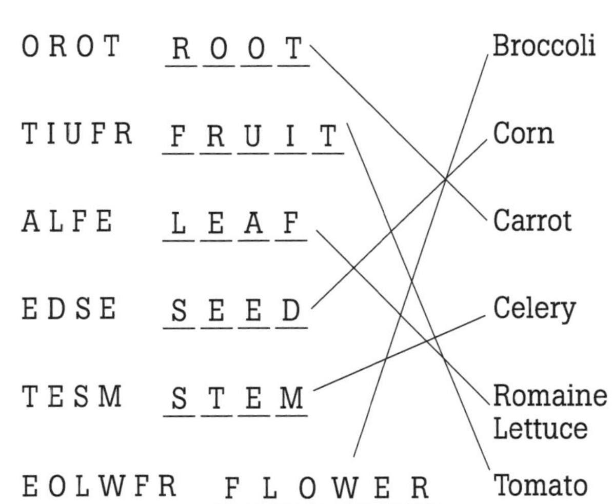

FRUIT: NATURE'S SWEET TREATS

Some fruits . . .

. . . grow on trees like these:

PAPELS A P P L E S
ECHPAES P E A C H E S
SRAEP P E A R S

. . . grow just fine on a vine:

PGARES G R A P E S
WIKIRTIUF K I W I F R U I T

. . . hang around on the ground:

TWMLAREEON W A T E R M E L O N
ENPPPAELI P I N E A P P L E
RBSWARTESIER S T R A W B E R R I E S

. . . feel pushed to hang on a bush:

SIRBUBLEERE B L U E B E R R I E S
RSBRISEREPA R A S P B E R R I E S

THE PROTEIN SCENE

1 EGGS
2 STRONG
3 DAIRY
4 PEANUT
4 PROTEIN
5 BEAN
6 FAT
7 FISH
8 GROW
9 SERVINGS

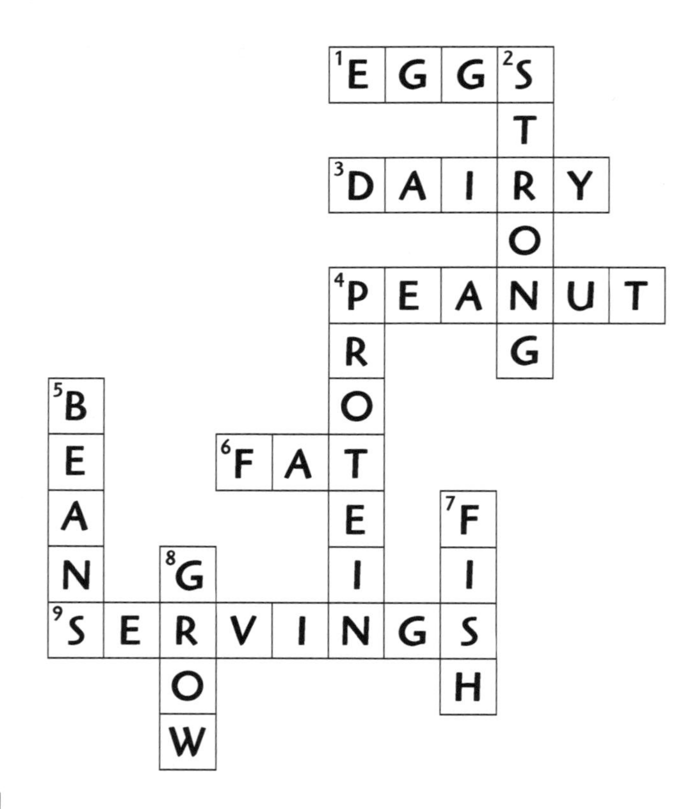

PUZZLE SOLUTIONS

USE YOUR BRAIN TO FIND WHOLE GRAINS!

Name ______________________________

"Your brain needs the energy from grains to solve this puzzle."

DIRECTIONS

Unscramble each whole grain food.
Then use the marked letters to solve the second puzzle.

OLAAEMT _ _ _ _ _ _ _ (1)

PRPOCON _ _ _ _ _ _ _ (8, 10)

BNWOR IRCE _ _ _ _ _   _ _ _ _ (11, 15, 13, 3)

WLHOE WEHAT EBDRA _ _ _ _ _   _ _ _ _ _   _ _ _ _ _ (16, 18, 19, 2, 12)

NBAR UMFNFI _ _ _ _   _ _ _ _ _ _ (5, 9, 7, 14)

WHLOE RCNO OTLTILRA _ _ _ _ _   _ _ _ _   _ _ _ _ _ _ _ _ (4, 17, 6)

_ _ k _   _ _ _ _   y _ _ _   g _ _ _ _ s   _ _ _ _ _ !

1 2   3   4 5 6 7   8 9 10   11 12 13 14   15 16 17 18 19

Word List: Bran Muffin, Brown Rice, Oatmeal, Popcorn ,Whole Corn Tortilla, Whole-Wheat Bread

WHOLE-GRAIN BLUEBERRY MUFFINS

Ingredients

1 cup fresh, frozen or canned blueberries, rinsed and drained
1-3/4 cups whole-wheat flour
1/2 cup sugar
2 teaspoons baking powder
2 eggs
8 oz. low-fat or fat-free lemon yogurt
1/4 cup canola oil
Non stick spray

Directions

Preheat oven to 375 degrees. Lightly spray muffin tin with non stick spray. Mix flour, sugar and baking powder in large mixing bowl. In another bowl, beat eggs and mix in yogurt and vegetable oil. Stir in dry ingredients and mix lightly. Fold in blueberries. Spoon batter into muffin cups. Bake 18–20 minutes or until muffin tops are browned. Loosen muffins and serve warm.

Makes 12 medium muffins

VEGGIE PLANT PARTS

Name ______________________________

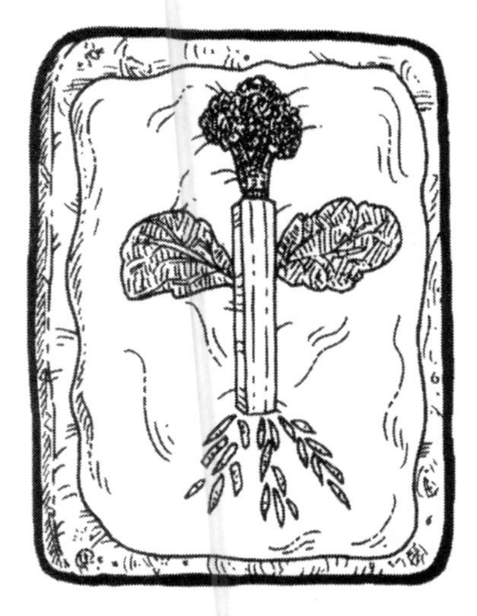

Did you know that vegetables come from all parts of the plant? Vegetables can be roots, stems, leaves, seeds, flowers or even fruit.*

DIRECTIONS

Unscramble the part of the plant on the left column. Next, draw a line from the plant part to the correct vegetable.

O R O T	_ _ _ _	Broccoli
T I U F R	_ _ _ _ _	Corn
A L F E	_ _ _ _	Carrot
E D S E	_ _ _ _	Celery
T E S M	_ _ _ _	Romaine Lettuce
E O L W F R	_ _ _ _ _ _	Tomato

WORD LIST: Flower, Fruit, Leaf, Root, Seed, Stem

**Yes, vegetables can actually be the "fruit" part of the plant. A botanist (a scientist who studies plants) classifies the fruit of the plant as the part that surrounds the seeds. Examples of vegetables that are the fruit part of the plant include zucchini, cucumbers, peppers, tomatoes and eggplant.*

PLANT PART ART

A Science Project You Can Eat!

Ingredients

- Large, flat cracker
- Peanut butter or low-fat cream cheese
- 2–3 broccoli florets
- 1 celery stick
- 1 lettuce leaf, torn into small pieces
- 1 T. grated carrots

Directions

Lightly spread cracker with either peanut butter or cream cheese. Next, create a plant or garden design on the cracker by arranging shredded carrots for roots, celery stick for the stem, lettuce for leaves and broccoli for flowers. EAT & ENJOY!

Serves 1

FRUIT: NATURE'S SWEET TREATS

Name ______________________________

"Fruit is a nutritious treat that is yummy-sweet. Fruits grow many different ways and in many different places."

DIRECTIONS

Unscramble the fruits to find out how they grow.

Some fruits . . .

. . . grow on trees like these:

PAPELS ___ ___ ___ ___ ___ ___

ECHPAES ___ ___ ___ ___ ___ ___ ___

SRAEP ___ ___ ___ ___ ___

. . . grow just fine on a vine:

PGARES ___ ___ ___ ___ ___ ___

WIKIRTIUF ___ ___ ___ ___ ___ ___ ___ ___ ___

. . . hang around on the ground:

TWMLAREEON ___ ___ ___ ___ ___ ___ ___ ___ ___ ___

ENPPPAELI ___ ___ ___ ___ ___ ___ ___ ___ ___

RBSWARTESIER ___ ___ ___ ___ ___ ___ ___ ___ ___ ___ ___ ___

. . . feel pushed to hang on a bush:

SIRBUBLEERE ___ ___ ___ ___ ___ ___ ___ ___ ___ ___ ___

RSBRISEREPA ___ ___ ___ ___ ___ ___ ___ ___ ___ ___ ___

WORD LIST: Apples, blueberries, grapes, kiwifruit, peaches, pears, pineapple, raspberries, strawberries, watermelon

MAKE-YOUR-OWN FRUIT KEBABS

Ingredients

Wooden skewers or plastic chopsticks
Different kinds of cut-up fruit (you choose!)
Whole berries and grapes
Low-fat or fat-free vanilla yogurt

Directions

Place fruit pieces on wooden skewers. Use your creativity to make beautiful designs and patterns! Dip in yogurt and eat. YUM!

THE PROTEIN SCENE

Name ______________________________

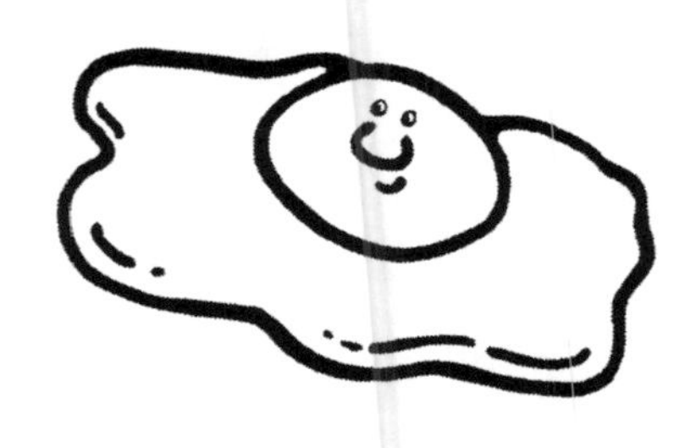

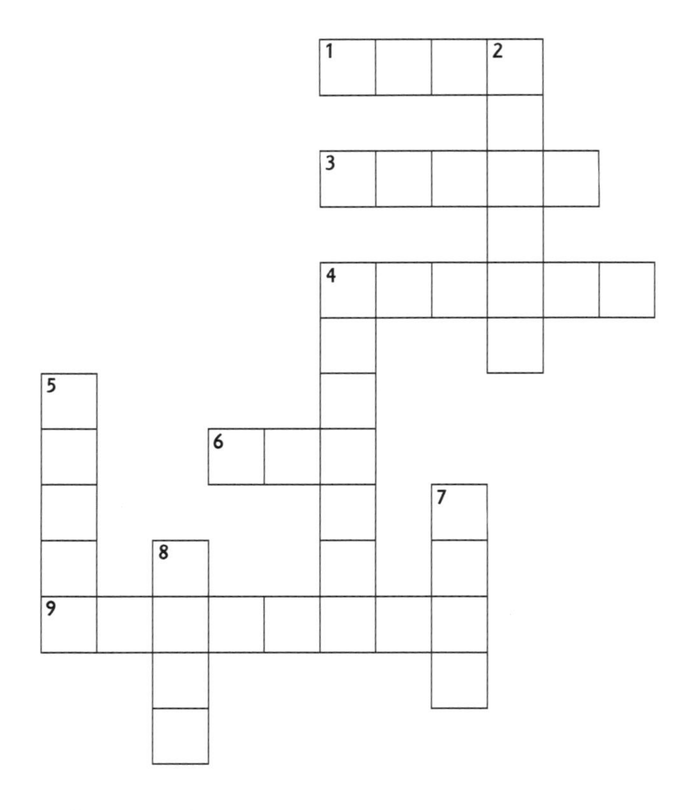

WORD LIST: Beans, Dairy, Eggs, Fat, Fish, Grow, Peanut, Protein, Servings, Strong

ACROSS:

1. Some kids like them scrambled.

3. Shown as a blue circle on *MyPlate*, this food group is also high in protein.

4. Grind this nut into butter for a popular sandwich filling.

6. Lean meats and chicken without skin are low in _ _ _

9. For good health, eat 4 to 6 ounces, or about 2–3 _ _ _ _ _ _ _ _ of protein-rich foods each day.

DOWN:

2. Foods from the Protein Group help to build a _ _ _ _ _ _ body.

4. A nutrient that provides the building blocks for growth.

5. Hugh-Man's favorite. You can find these in burritos.

7. A protein food that lives in the water.

8. Get bigger.

EASY LENTIL CHILI

This recipe can be served as a thick, hearty soup, as a filling for tortillas or as a topping for baked potatoes.

Ingredients

1 pound lentils, rinsed
5 cups water
1 can tomato sauce (15 oz.)
1/2 cup chopped onion
3 teaspoons chili powder
1/2 teaspoon salt (optional)
1 cup grated cheddar cheese

Directions

Combine lentils and water in a large pan. Place on the stove and bring to a boil. Turn the heat down, cover with a lid and simmer for 30 minutes. Add tomato sauce, onion, chili powder and salt. Simmer for 30 minutes more. Top each serving bowl with 2 tablespoons of grated cheddar cheese.

Makes 6–8 servings

A *M-O-O-O-O-VING* STORY ABOUT DAIRY

Name ______________________________

DIRECTIONS

1. Answer the questions below.
2. Use the words from this page to fill in the story on page 62.

Note: No peeking at the story before you answer the questions!

Name a type of truck ______________________________
A

Favorite variety of cheese ______________________________
B

Your best friend's name ______________________________
C

Favorite animal ______________________________
D

Favorite sport ______________________________
E

Name a material that is very hard ______________________________
F

Favorite holiday ______________________________
G

The type of milk that you usually drink ______________________________
H

Favorite song ______________________________
I

The month of your birthday ______________________________
J

Town where you live ______________________________
K

Favorite color ______________________________
L

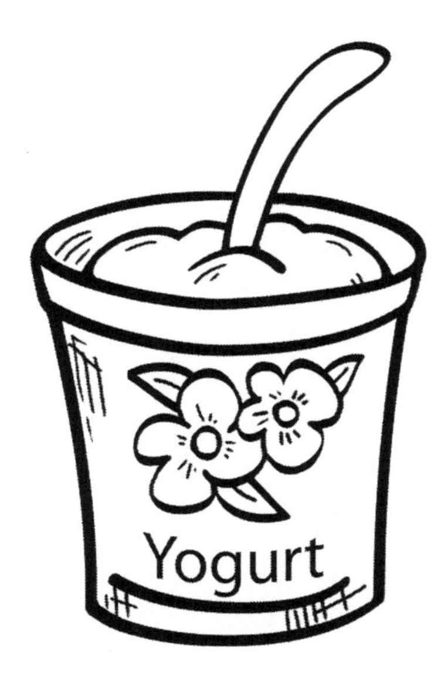

BANANA SMOOTHIE

Ingredients

1 banana, peeled and frozen
3/4 cup low-fat milk
1/2 cup low-fat vanilla yogurt
1/4 cup orange juice

Directions

Place ingredients in blender. Blend until smooth and creamy. Serve chilled.
Makes 2 servings

Suggested Level: 1st - 6th grade

A *M-O-O-O-O-VING* STORY ABOUT DAIRY

Name ______________________________

Cruising along in my ______________________________ on the narrow, winding roads of
A

Mount ______________________, I suddenly came across a ______________________ cow.
B L

Right beside her was a ______________________, singing ______________________ as loudly
D I

as he could. When the ________________________ saw me, he stopped, stared at me for a
D

moment and asked me what I was carrying in my ______________________.
A

I replied, "I have a load of dairy products that I'm delivering to ______________________,
K

just in time for the ________________________ celebration. Did you know that those
G

folks always celebrate ________________________ in ________________________?"
G J

The cow, who introduced herself as __________________________, was very pleased that
C

I was carrying ________________________ milk, yogurt and cheese in my truck. She asked
H

me if I knew why dairy products were important for good health.

The __________________________ interrupted, anxious to tell me that dairy foods have a
D

lot of calcium, a nutrient that makes bones as strong as ________________________.
F

__________________________ agreed and also mentioned that you need strong bones to do
C

your best at __________________________.
E

After a snack of crackers, grapes and __________________________, I said good-bye and
B

rushed along on my way to __________________________, delivering my goods just in
K

time for __________________________.
G

Suggested Level: 1st - 6th grade

A MONTH OF FITNESS & FUN!

Name ______________________________

Month ______________________________

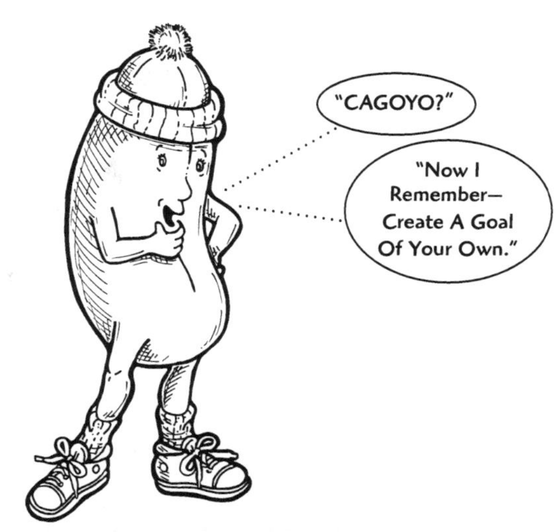

DIRECTIONS

Mark an "**X**" in the square for each day that you complete the suggested activity.

SUN	MON	TUE	WED	THU	FRI	SAT
Discover a new place that your family can hike.	Walk your dog for at least 20 minutes. No dog? No problem. Walk your neighbor's or friend's dog.	Read a book about healthy eating.*	Click on choosemyplate.gov to learn more about the food groups and what your body needs.	CAGOYO	Put video games on "pause" today. Instead, ask a friend to ride bikes together.	Plan next week's breakfast menus. Include three different food groups in each plan.
Set up an aerobic obstacle course in your yard or play area.	Visit *kidshealth.org* and click on the "kids" site. It is packed with games, trivia, recipes and videos!	Play street hockey with your friends using brooms and a tennis ball.	CAGOYO	Create a commercial for a healthy food. Perform for your friends, classmates, family or a video camera.	Try a new fruit or vegetable today.	Look in the library or bookstore for fun and healthy kids' cookbooks.
Grab some sidewalk chalk and draw the "world's longest hopscotch game" down your sidewalk. See how many spaces you can hop!	Put on your chef's hat and help make dinner tonight.	CAGOYO	Make up a new recipe for your after-school snack today.	Visit *foodchamps.org* for fun fruit and veggie recipes, activities and games.	Play **"Don't Laugh"** with your friends. Sit in a circle and take turns saying "Don't laugh." The game is over when everyone is laughing!	Create a piñata shaped like a fruit or vegetable. Fill it with healthy prizes.
Use cookie cutters to cut pancakes or waffles into fun shapes. Serve with berries and low-fat yogurt.	Write a story or poem about healthy food and fun activity.	Turn off the TV and play an active game after school today.	Visit *kidnetic.com* for fun ideas on how to move more.	Try a new grain today. (How about quinoa, couscous millet or bulgur?)	CAGOYO	Look through gardening catalogs, and pick out a new vegetable to grow.

***Reading about eating ideas:**

Good for You! Nutrition Book and Games, by Connie Evers, Disney Learning, 2006.

Janey Junkfood's fresh adventure! Making Good Eating Great Fun! by Barbara Storper, FoodPlay Productions, 2011.

The ABCs of fruits and vegetables and beyond, by Steve Charney & David Goldbeck, Ceres Press, 2007.

Suggested Level: 1st - 6th grade

It's Hugh-Man
(and the Foodettes)

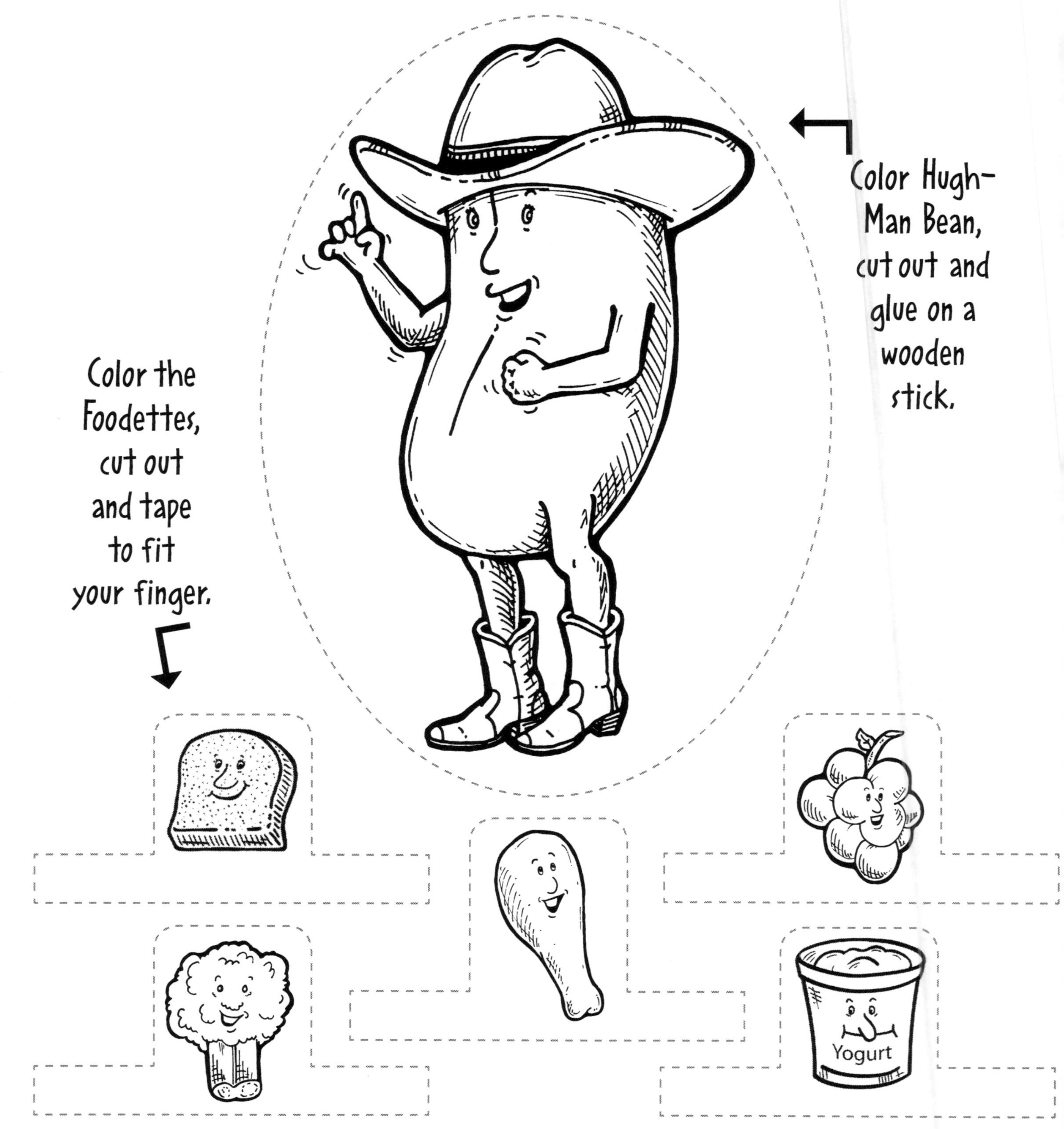

Suggested Level: K-2nd grade

Made in the USA
Charleston, SC
31 May 2012